DRUGS AND AGING

by

William A. McKim
Psychology Department and Gerontology Centre
Memorial University of Newfoundland,

and

Brian L. Mishara
Psychology Department
Université du Québec à Montréal

Butterworths
Toronto and Vancouver

Drugs and Aging
English language edition © 1987 Butterworths, A division of Reed Inc.

Printed and bound in Canada

The Butterworth Group of Companies
Canada
Butterworths, Toronto and Vancouver
United Kingdom
Butterworth & Co. (Publishers) Ltd., London and Edinburgh
Australia
Butterworth Pty Ltd., Sydney, Melbourne, Brisbane, Adelaide and Perth
New Zealand
Butterworths (New Zealand) Ltd., Wellington and Auckland
Singapore
Butterworth & Co. (Asia) Pte. Ltd., Singapore
South Africa
Butterworth Publishers (SA) (Pty) Ltd., Durban and Pretoria
United States
Butterworth Legal Publishers, Boston, Seattle, Austin and St. Paul
D&S Publishers, Clearwater

Canadian Cataloguing in Publication Data

McKim, William A., 1945-
  Drugs and Aging

(Perspectives on individual and population aging)
Bibliography: p.
Includes index.
ISBN 0-409-80517-3

1. Geriatric pharmacology.   2. Aged – Drug use.
I. Mishara, Brian L.   II. Title.   III. Series.

RC953.7.M24 1987   615.5'47   C87-093648-4

Executive Editor (P. & A.): Lebby Hines
Sponsoring Editor: Janet Turner
Managing Editor: Linda Kee
Supervisory Editor: Marie Graham
Freelance Projects Coordinator: Joan Chaplin
Editor: Maura Brown
Cover Design: Patrick Ng
Production: Jill Thomson

BUTTERWORTHS PERSPECTIVES ON INDIVIDUAL AND POPULATION AGING SERIES

The initiation of this Series represents an exciting and significant development for gerontology in Canada. Since the production of Canadian-based knowledge about individual and population aging is expanding rapidly, students, scholars and practitioners are seeking comprehensive yet succinct summaries of the literature on specific topics. Recognizing the common need of this diverse community of gerontologists, Janet Turner, Sponsoring Editor at Butterworths, conceived the idea of a series of specialized monographs that could be used in gerontology courses to complement existing texts and, at the same time, to serve as a valuable reference for those initiating research, developing policies, or providing services to elderly Canadians.

Each monograph includes a state-of-the-art review and analysis of the Canadian-based scientific and professional knowledge on the topic. Where appropriate for comparative purposes, information from other countries is introduced. In addition, some important policy and program implications of the current knowledge base are discussed, and unanswered policy and research questions are raised to stimulate further work in the area. The monographs have been written for a wide audience: undergraduate students in a variety of gerontology courses; graduate students and research personnel who need a summary and analysis of the Canadian literature prior to initiating research projects; practitioners who are involved in the daily planning and delivery of services to aging adults; and policy-makers who require current and reliable information in order to design, implement and evaluate policies and legislation for an aging population.

The decision to publish a monograph on a specific topic has been based in part on the relevance of the topic for the academic and professional community, as well as on the extent of information available at the time an author is signed to a contract. Thus, not all the conceivable topics are included in the early stages of the Series and some topics are published earlier rather than later. Because gerontology in Canada is attracting large numbers of highly qualified graduate students as well as increasingly active research personnel in academic, public and private settings, new areas of concentrated research will evolve. Hence, additional monographs that review and analyze work in these areas will be needed to reflect the evolution of knowledge on specialized topics pertaining to individual or population aging in Canada.

Before introducing the third monograph in the Series, I would like, on behalf of the Series' authors and the gerontology community, to acknowledge the following members of the Butterworths "team" and their respective staffs for their unique and sincere contribution to gerontology in Canada: Geoffrey Burn, President, for his continuing support of the project despite difficult times in the Canadian publishing industry; Janet Turner, Sponsoring Editor, for her vision, endurance and high academic standards; Linda Kee, Managing Editor, for her coordination of the production, especially her constant reminders to authors (and the Series Editor) that the hands of the clock continue to move in spite of our perceptions that manuscript deadlines were still months or years away; Jim Shepherd, Production Manager, for nimbly vaulting many a technical obstacle; and Gloria Vitale, Academic Sales Manager, for her support and promotion of the Series. For each of you, we hope the knowledge provided in this Series will have personal value — but not until well into the next century!

Barry D. McPherson
Series Editor

FOREWORD

Unlike the first two monographs in the Series, wherein the focus was on population aging (*Canada's Aging Population* and *Aging and Ethnicity*), in this monograph and the next (Brillon, *Victimization and Fear of Crime Among The Elderly*) the emphasis is on the aging individual. However, even though the major focus in any given monograph is on individual or population aging, there is considerable interaction between the two levels. To illustrate, most of the attention in this monograph is on the use of drugs by aging individuals. Nevertheless, the patterns of individual use are influenced by societal norms and values, and by policies concerning the availability and consumption of drugs. For example, the prescription practices of physicians, the availability of private and public sector drug plans, and the amount of knowledge about drug interactions and age-related changes in the sensitivity to drugs are all related to drug use, abuse, or non-compliance among older adults.

Increasingly, the use of drugs to maintain or enhance the health and activity level of aging adults has become a prevalent practice. As shown in this monograph, the elderly receive more prescribed drugs and purchase more over-the-counter medication than any other age group. As a result, the misuse or abuse of drugs among the elderly population is a potential problem. While the extent and severity of this problem is not well documented, an increasing number of drug-related concerns are being identified and reported by relatives, by health-care workers, and by social workers. Furthermore, our awareness of the issue is heightened when extreme cases of abuse or misuse are dramatically portrayed by the media when the outcome leads to sudden hospitalization, or death. Some frequently reported examples of non-compliance or abuse include: hoarding drugs and using drugs beyond the expiry date; purchasing an extra supply of a specific drug or more than one drug after receiving prescriptions from more than one physician; using a mixture of prescribed and over-the-counter drugs; exchanging drugs with another person; misinterpreting label instructions or misidentifying drugs on a shelf; failing to consume drugs on schedule or with appropriate liquids or foods; and, because of physical limitations, being unable to open drug containers. Moreover, these self-induced problems can be heightened or compounded by the prescribing practices of physicians, or by inappropriate advice from a friend, relative, or professional care-giver.

This monograph, written for professionals (nurses, social workers, physicians, pharmacists, gerontology students, and researchers), as well as older adults and their relatives, sensitizes the reader to age-related changes in the use, effects, and potential misuse of drugs. These age-related processes and problems are discussed from a social science rather than a medical or pharmacological perspective. Throughout, Professors McKim and Mishara emphasize the importance of considering individual differences in the use and effects of drugs that are associated with physiological, anatomical, or health changes that accompany aging. We also learn that these individual differences can be influenced by cohort or history effects, by sociodemographic factors (*e.g.*, gender, class, ethnicity, and education), or by dietary or alcohol consumption patterns that change with age.

In Chapter 1, key concepts for understanding the interaction of drug use and individual aging are defined, and in Chapter 2 the reader is introduced to pharmacokinetics — the study of the processes of drug ingestion, absorption, distribution, and elimination. To illustrate, we learn that age-related physiological and anatomical changes in the proportion of body fat can alter the effectiveness and the effect of some drugs. This chapter also describes age-related changes in drug interactions and drug sensitivity, both of which can contribute to the increasing heterogeneity among older adults in their responses to a given drug, or to a combination of drugs.

Chapter 3, illustrated with considerable Canadian data, describes the pattern of increased use, and increased multiple use, of drugs with advancing age. This pattern is especially pronounced for women, and it cannot be explained merely by the fact that there are more women living to an older age. Rather, research has shown that this gender difference in drug use begins in early adulthood. The authors also discuss how a number of psychological and sociological factors are related to patterns of drug use in the later years, and why there may be varying degrees of drug compliance among the elderly.

In the next two chapters the authors consider possible influences that may increase drug use during the middle and later years. First, Chapter 4 draws upon various theories of aging to describe historical and contemporary attempts by aging adults to use drugs, special diets or alterations in lifestyle in an effort to either preserve or restore youth, or to prolong life. Then, in Chapter 5 the use and effects of recreational drugs (substances consumed for non-medical reasons) to alter experiences or to cope more successfully with life are discussed. This chapter also identifies the use, side-effects, and addiction rates among the elderly for substances such as caffeine, tobacco, alcohol, and some psychoactive drugs.

The final two chapters examine the need for prevention, intervention, research, and policies concerning drug use and abuse in middle and later adulthood. Chapter 6 describes the primary, secondary, and tertiary levels of prevention and intervention that can be used for various types of drug problems, and analyzes two current problems: alcoholism among native people and the alleviation of pain in the terminally ill patient. As in all monographs in the Series, the final chapter proposes an agenda for research and policy directions that are needed in Canada.

In conclusion, like elder abuse, we do not know fully the extent to which drug abuse or misuse occurs, or why it occurs only among some elderly adults. Nevertheless, our understanding and level of awareness of this potential problem is significantly enhanced by this monograph. Specifically, factual information is provided about the use and misuse by older adults of prescribed, over-the-counter, and recreational drugs. Based on this current knowledge, effective programs and policies to educate older adults, to insure compliance, and to prevent abuse or misuse can be designed and implemented. Furthermore, the basic information and unanswered research questions introduced in the monograph should stimulate scholars in a number of disciplines to engage in further basic, applied, and policy research concerning drugs and aging in Canada.

Barry D. McPherson, Ph.D.
Series Editor
Waterloo, Ontario, Canada
March, 1987

PREFACE

The use of drugs has become an increasingly important aspect of the lives and health of older people in Canada. While the use of recreational drugs shows a decline with age, older people in our society consume a disproportionately large amount of prescribed and non-prescribed medicines. At the same time they have altered sensitivities to drugs, are more susceptible to the adverse effects of many drugs, and are more likely to use medicines incorrectly. Because these age-related changes are not well understood, the problems they create are frequently not identified correctly and are left untreated or, worse still, treated inappropriately. For example, the symptoms of senile dementia are similar to the symptoms caused by overuse of sedatives or antipsychotic drugs. In treating such symptoms the correct response should be a decrease in drugs, but frequently the dose and the number of prescribed drugs are increased in response to these symptoms, thus exacerbating the problem and robbing the older person and his or her family of significant and valuable interactions and life experiences. This book is for both professionals and non-professionals who work with older people, for students of gerontology with a variety of backgrounds, for families of older people, and for older people themselves. This book is for all those who are in a position to recognize and prevent such tragedies. Furthermore, we believe this book will be of interest to medical, pharmacological, and mental health professionals who do not specialize in gerontology, but feel that they should be informed about the important issues concerning drugs and the older person.

In this book we review the classical and current literature on drug use by older people, defining our topic in a rather broad manner so as to include recreational drugs like caffeine and alcohol in addition to medicines. This has been done with two constraints. The first is that we do not assume the reader has a background in gerontology or pharmacology. Consequently, we have attempted to avoid the use of jargon wherever possible, and where this has been impossible, we have tried to provide a non-technical explanation of the terms we used. We have also supplied a glossary at the end of the book to provide a quick reference to many key terms.

We believe this book can be understood by anyone interested in the area, whether or not they have an extensive medical, psychological, or pharmacological background. This is not to say that this book is inappropriate for physicians, psychologists, pharmacists, and nurses. Such professionals are often in need of a better understanding of the problems that older people have with drugs. Such a lack of understanding on the part of many professionals seems to be at the root of many problems older people have with drugs. While those with medical training may find some of the material presented here oversimplified, we believe that the issues we discuss and the data we present will be both informative and useful to any highly trained medical or behavioural professional.

Secondly, there are constraints on the length of this book which have prevented us from presenting an exhaustive review of all published material in the area. The studies we discuss are representative rather than exhaustive. Other considerations being equal, we have included material from Canadian sources about Canadians whenever this has been possible. Our aim has not been to describe Canadians and Canadian problems exclusively; the problems and solutions discussed here are typical of all Western industrialized countries. Whenever possible we have tried to go beyond simple presentation of the relevant information and have sought to understand the implications of the current state of knowledge for improved professional practices, better and more appropriate government policies, and more informed individual decisions about drugs, all of which, we hope, will improve the quality of the lives of older people.

We would like to acknowledge the valuable assistance of the following people who have helped us at various stages of the preparation of the manuscript: Lisa Brake, Valarie Davie, Michael Stones, Ken Roberts, Ed Napke, and François Labelle, who drew the figures.

W.A.M.
St. John's
B.L.M.
Montréal
September 30, 1986

CONTENTS

TABLES

FIGURES

CHAPTER 1

INTRODUCTION

It is usual at the beginning of a book of this nature to define the terms that are going to be used and to introduce the reader to the approach that the authors have taken toward their material. Since this book is on the use of drugs by older people, it is probably a good idea to start with a brief discussion of what we mean by some of the words we will be using. There is also a glossary in the back of the book that will give much briefer definitions for quick reference.

DRUG

"Drug" is used by different writers in many different ways to suit their own prejudices and biases. In addition, different professions may mean something different when they use the term (Napke 1983, p. XIX). This makes it an extremely difficult concept to pin down with any precision. In this book we will be talking about a variety of substances of diverse nature and have decided that the simplest approach is not to define the word at all, apart from saying that we consider a drug to be anything that we talk about in these pages. However, we do feel that some discussion of the term is warranted.

The term "drug" was originally used to identify a substance by its form. The word is derived from the old French "drogue" meaning a dry powder. Such a description is of no use today because drugs come in solid, liquid, and gaseous form, but in this sense the word drug also implies a certain degree of refinement or purity of the substance which in its purest form is frequently a dry powder. It is easy to find obvious exceptions to this type of definition. A drug like caffeine is almost always consumed in the unrefined form of coffee or tea, and the nicotine in tobacco has never been consumed in concentrated form (at least until the invention of nicotine gum). Nonetheless, we can still understand the effects of these substances in terms of their single active ingredient.

A substance is often defined as a drug in terms of the particular purposes for which it might be taken, *i.e.*, drugs are substances that are used to treat disease or to make a person high. This type of definition, however, presents us with many problems, not the least of which is that we do not really understand why any drug is consumed. Tobacco was used by South American Indians to create hallucinations and to contact the spirits of the departed; in Europe in the seventeenth century it was used for protection from the plague and today may well be used by young people to make them look grown up (McKim 1986). In addition, our perceptions of why a drug is being used can be coloured by prejudices and cultural beliefs and practices. For example, it has only been in recent years that we have come to describe tobacco smoking and alcohol consumption as forms of drug taking. Prior to that, these activities were so common that their similarity to heroin use and smoking of marijuana was not understood. It is obviously inappropriate to define what a drug is in terms of why we think people take it.

In a functional sense, we might well describe a drug as a substance that interacts with the physiological processes of the body. This is a fairly good definition except that it seems to include substances that we normally call food. An orange is a substance that interacts with the body in several ways, two of which are by (a) providing sugar that the body uses for energy and (b) providing vitamin C which is vital to the normal metabolism of the body. An orange is a food, not a drug. One could argue that if we extract and refine the vitamin C and give it separately then it is a drug. Strangely enough this sort of argument is seldom made for sugar.

If this discussion has served no other purpose it illustrates why we do not bother to define the term at all, apart from saying that a drug is whatever we decide to talk about in this book. Generally, we have taken a rather broad view and decided to include substances such as alcohol, coffee, and tobacco, often described as recreational drugs, and drugs usually described as medicines, including over-the-counter medicines (OTC) and drugs prescribed by a physician.

DRUG NAMES

In addition to the confusion created by the many definitions of the word "drug," there is a further source of confusion created by the way drugs are named. Drugs sold as medicines have two types of names, generic and trade names. The generic name refers to the active ingredient of a medicine and is not capitalized, while the trade name refers to a specific preparation of that active ingredient sold by a particular manufacturer and is always capitalized. For example, diazepam is the generic name of a drug sold under the trade name of Valium by Hoffman-LaRoche Ltd. The same substance, diazepam, is also sold in Canada as Vivol by Frank W. Horner Ltd., and Novodiapam by Novopharm Ltd. It is sold under seven other trade names in Canada and many more in the United States and other countries. In addition, it may also be sold under the generic name of diazepam. While all the preparations of diazepam contain diazepam, they are not necessarily all the same. They may differ in the type of other ingredients that they are mixed with. These other substances are called excipients and are added for such purposes as binding, diluting, lubrication, colouring and flavouring. They are supposed to be inert and have no effect, but many do (Napke 1983). In this book we will adhere to the practice of referring to drugs by their generic names, although in some cases we will also give the most common trade name used in this country. While we will be treating all preparations that contain that substance as though they were the same, it is important to keep in mind that this may not always be the case.

DRUG DEPENDENCE

There are several other concepts that should also be considered at this time. One of them is drug dependence. This is probably the most misused and misunderstood term in the entire field of pharmacology. The main problem is that the word is all too often used as an explanation of drug taking. In reality, it does not explain anything, it just describes what is going on. The term "physical" or "physiological dependence" should only be used to describe the state where the discontinuation of a regularly administered drug causes physiological changes known as withdrawal symptoms. It is assumed all too often that physical dependence on a drug is the sole reason why people continue to take it. In reality, most research has shown that physical dependence is only a contributory factor in the self-administration of drugs, and the concept cannot be used as an explanation of drug taking in general. Thus, to say that someone is physically dependent on a drug should only suggest that withdrawal symptoms will follow if the drug is discontinued. It is not an explanation of why the drug is self-administered on a regular basis.

The term "psychological dependence" also deserves some comment. It has been known for some time that many self-administered drugs produce virtually no physical withdrawal symptoms. This has caused problems for those who assume that the main motive for continuing to use a drug is fear of withdrawal. In order to reconcile this fact it was suggested that self-administered drugs that caused minimal or no physical withdrawal symptoms did cause psychological withdrawal symptoms that motivated the use of these drugs. Hence the term "psychological dependence." As well, we should be careful not to be misled by this term for two reasons. First, like physical dependence, there is little evidence that withdrawal of any kind really can explain drug taking. Second, the existence of psychological dependence is frequently inferred only from the presence of drug taking. This leads to a tautology, *i.e.*, the drug taking is explained by the state of "psychological dependence" and the only evidence that there is psychological dependence is the drug taking.

For all the above reasons, the term "dependence" presents similar difficulties. To avoid some of these we have adopted a very simple behavioural definition first suggested by Thompson and Schuster in their book *Behavioral Pharmacology* (1968). They suggested that dependence be defined as "the repeated and reliable self-administration of a drug." This permits us to describe a state of affairs without suggesting any explanation. Such a description allows us to consider a wide variety of behaviour under the description of "dependence"; behaviours ranging from shooting up heroin to sipping a glass of wine with meals, to the daily injection of insulin. Admittedly these behaviours appear to be quite different from the perspective of our culture and time. This definiton forces us to concede that all these behaviours are similar enough to be considered as drug dependence and permits us to entertain the possibility that all of these acts may well be under the control of similar environmental and behavioural factors. Taking such a broad definition also forces us to be non-judgmental and make no presumptions about the value of the activity. Drug taking has both benefits and costs. No drug is entirely without benefit or cost, and judgments about the goodness or dangers of a drug must be made within a personal, emotional, medical, social, and cultural context.

Thus, in this book we recognize the term "dependence" to mean "the repeated and reliable self-administration of a drug." "Physical dependence," on the other hand, refers to the state where the discontinuation of a drug will cause an identifiable set of physiological changes called "withdrawal symptoms." The two terms "physical dependence" and "dependence" are quite different and should not be interchanged.

CONCEPTS OF AGING

What do we mean by "older people"? Mishara and Riedel (1984) distinguish between chronological age, physiological and biological age, psychological and emotional age, and social age. Someone may be chronologically over 70, but have a body whose biological aging and health status is equivalent to that of another person 20 years younger. Similarly, a person who is only 40 years of age may be physically deteriorated due to disease and abuse, and physically resemble a person who is much older. For example, some authors feel that alcohol abuse early in life produces premature aging at the physical and biological levels.

Psychological and emotional age refers to levels of "maturity," cognitive capacities, wisdom, etc. Social age concerns roles people have in society and how people are viewed and treated in society as a result of their age.

In current gerontology research it is widely accepted that simple chronological age criteria are not adequate to describe the complex processes involved in aging. Various measures of functional aging have been used to compensate partially for the problems involved in the use of chronological age to classify, understand, and predict behaviour. Unfortunately, current research on drugs and older people has not yet used such measures of functional age. Most studies simply choose an arbitrary chronological age cut-off point for classifying persons as "elderly," or not. Therefore, in this book we are obliged to use such chronological criteria to define what we mean by "older people." We report on whatever definitions of "old" or "elderly" researchers have used in the studies we report. However, we do so with an awareness of the fact that "old," in terms of number of years since birth, is a crude generalization which overlooks the richness of individual differences in aging processes at the physical and biological, psychological and emotional, and social levels.

In this book we try to go beyond simple generalizations about differences between the "young" and the "old" by discussing processes rather than just age differences. We try to understand which processes can account for observed age differences. For example, age differences in levels of blood alcohol in persons of equivalent weight who have consumed the same amount of alcohol are probably due to typical age changes in the percentage of lean body mass in the body. Bodies tend to have a greater percentage of fat as they grow older, and it is probably this process that explains many age differences in drinking behaviour and in blood alcohol levels that occur with age. (See Chapter 2.)

An important consideration in any work on aging is the distinction between processes which are age-related and processes or changes which are (1) attributable to the generation or cohort a person was born into and (2) effects due to the year of measurement — historical changes due to the time the research was conducted. People who were born and raised at the beginning of this century are different from people in more recent generations due to differences in education, social values, life experiences, eating habits, etc. These "cohort" differences may explain many findings that show differences in people of different ages. For example, the fact that older people do not use much marijuana and certain other recreational drugs may simply reflect the fact that these drugs were not a part of their experiences early in life. When the generation of Canadians who currently use these recreational drugs more frequently becomes old, they may very well continue their relatively high level of recreational drug use. In this instance we are observing cohort differences which do not reflect changes related to aging as such. In many cases, unfortunately, it is not possible to determine at this point whether an age difference is due to cohort or other effects.

Despite long entrenched patterns of drug use due to cohort differences, certain drug-use patterns change with age. For example, several studies report that people often reduce their consumption of alcohol and cigarettes due to a concern for their health as they grow older (See Chapter 5). In addition, the time when a study is conducted is also an important factor to consider, since certain drug-use practices are more prevalent at certain times in history. Heroin was as easy to obtain as aspirin at the turn of the century and was regarded at that time as being as safe as aspirin to use. Studies of drug use at that time may have come to completely different conclusions than contemporary research. More recently, certain drugs like the benzodiazepines (Librium and Valium) are "in vogue" and are widely used and prescribed for older people. In five or ten years these may be seen as less desirable and new drugs may take their place. Conclusions drawn about these drugs in the 1980s may not apply in the 1990s.

When we discuss research in this book, we try to distinguish between differences which may be related to the processes of aging, age-group differences which are more likely due to cohort differences, and transitory differences due to the year when the investigation took place. We present the current state of knowledge on the use of drugs by older people. However, we are aware that future generations may be different from the present generation of older Canadians. Hence the drug-use patterns and potential drug problems of the elderly in the future may be different from the present due to changes in society or to changes in beliefs and practices relating to drug use.

CHAPTER 2

AGE-RELATED CHANGES IN ABSORPTION, DISTRIBUTION, EXCRETION AND SENSITIVITY TO DRUGS

INTRODUCTION

Before any drug can have an effect, it must get from outside the body to a particular place inside the body, known as the site of action, where it alters the body's physiology. For example, tranquilizers must reach specific sites in the brain before they can tranquilize. Generally, the extent of the effect of a drug is determined by how much of it gets to the site of action. It is, therefore, important to understand the mechanisms involved in getting the drug to and from the site of action in order to understand how these mechanisms can influence its effect. The term "pharmacokinetics," which literally means "movement of drugs," refers to the study of these processes. It is especially important to understand pharmacokinetics in order to have a reasonable understanding of how aging changes our response to drugs, because many of the physiological and anatomical changes that occur as we age alter the pharmacokinetics of drugs, and consequently, their effect.

ABSORPTION

Most drugs are taken orally; they are swallowed and pass through the stomach and intestines and if they are not absorbed, they are eliminated with the feces. Drugs are seldom absorbed to any extent directly from the stomach. Instead they are absorbed through the walls of the intestine, which are designed for the purpose of extracting nutrients from our food. Blood flows in large quantities near the inside surface of the intestine and carries the drug absorbed through the intestine wall throughout the body. Before a drug can get to the intestine, however, it must first pass through the stomach, and so the functioning of the stomach is capable of influencing absorption from the intestine in several ways.

If the stomach contents enter the intestine slowly, blood levels of the drug will rise slowly, never reaching very high levels, and the drug effect will have a long duration. If a drug passes through the stomach quickly, it will have a high peak level in the blood and short duration. For some individuals, aging causes a decrease in the rate of passage through the stomach which reduces the speed of absorption of drugs taken orally. Apart from this direct effect of age on stomach emptying, there are a number of second-ary age-related changes that can delay drug absorption. These include erratic eating habits, changes in diet, inadequate fluid intake, states of anxi-ety and depression and the presence of other drugs such as antacids and laxatives. All these factors can alter the functioning of the digestive system and change absorption of drugs in unpredictable ways.

In addition to delayed digestion in the stomach, the acidity of the stomach can influence the degree to which the molecules of a drug become ionized or carry an electric charge. Ionized molecules are water soluble and will dissolve readily in the contents of the digestive system, but they are not lipid soluble and this means that they are unable to pass through the mem-branes of the intestine wall into the blood. (Fat tissue is composed of lipid molecules, and drugs that are lipid soluble will dissolve in body fat. Mem-branes of the body are also made up of lipid molecules so a drug must be lipid soluble in order to pass through membranes). Achlorhydria is an age-related condition where the acidity of the stomach is reduced (Vanzant *et al.* 1932). This has the effect of changing the ionization and differentially decreasing the rate of absorption of drugs like aspirin, which are weak acids that are not normally ionized in the intestine, and increasing absorption of weak bases like morphine, which are normally more highly ionized. In addition to natural achlorhydria, some over-the-counter drugs like antacids also reduce stomach acidity and can have the same effect. As we shall dis-cuss in Chapter 3, people tend to consume more antacids as they get older (See Figure 3.1), and this increased consumption of antacids may have important implications for understanding the effects of other drugs.

While ionization decreases lipid solubility, it increases water solubility and, consequently, the ability of a drug to dissolve in the contents of the digestive system, a step that must take place before any drug can be absorbed. This tends to speed absorption. Changes in the acidity of the stomach can also alter the rate at which tablets disintegrate. In fact, some tablets require an acidic environment before they will even dissolve (Bates *et al.* 1974). Such tablets would be of little value to someone with decreased stomach acidity as a result of achlorhydria or excessive use of antacids.

There are also a number of age-related changes in the intestine that can influence absorption. In general, because of decreases in the tone and strength of the muscles in the intestine wall, the rate of passage of food through the intestine is decreased. This has the effect of increasing the length of time a drug is available for absorption.

While all these changes suggest that there should be significant alterations in drug absorption in older people, many studies have shown no actual age-related difference between the young and the elderly in the amount of drug absorbed. However, those studies that do show age-related effects find these changes are largely reflected in a slowing of the rate of absorption of many drugs with age (Mayersohn 1982).

So far, we have dealt with absorption of drugs after oral administration, but drugs can also be administered by other routes such as by injection, absorption from mucous membranes like those under the tongue or in the nose, or by inhalation. There is no research on age-related changes in absorption from these sites, but it might be reasonable to speculate that absorption from these areas might also be slower in older people. Absorption depends upon blood flow to the area where the drug is applied, and since total cardiac output diminishes with age, it is likely that there is diminished absorption from all sites in the elderly (Mayersohn 1982). This is clearly an area where more research is needed.

DISTRIBUTION

Once a drug has been absorbed into the blood, it is distributed around the body and is absorbed differentially by different organs and tissues. This process is known as drug distribution. As described earlier, drugs differ in their preference for being dissolved in lipids (fats) or water. Lipid soluble drugs will tend to become concentrated in body fat and water soluble drugs will dissolve in body water. There are definite changes with age in the percent of body fat and water and these changes alter the distribution of drugs in older people.

Figure 2.1 (Forbes and Reina 1970) shows age-related changes in lean body mass and fat body mass for both men and women. It is clear from this figure that for men there is a significant decline in lean body mass and an increase in the proportion of body fat. The same changes take place with women, but since women have a larger percentage of body fat to begin with, these changes are not as dramatic. This change in body composition is important in determining the distribution of drugs. Lipid soluble drugs like the barbiturates tend to be absorbed by the increased body fat of older people and reach lower concentrations in the rest of the body, including the blood. On the other hand, drugs like alcohol that are distributed primarily to body water reach higher concentrations in the blood of an older person because they will be distributed throughout a smaller volume. This means that an older person needs to drink less alcohol to achieve the same blood level as a younger person of equal size. Because of the greater proportion of body fat in women, women have always been more sensitive to alcohol than men, and the change with age is less dramatic in women than in men. Men experience a much greater increase in sensitivity to alcohol and other water soluble drugs as they age.

Another age-related change in drug distribution is protein binding. Once in the blood, molecules of many drugs become bound to large protein molecules (usually albumen). Because of their size, these proteins cannot leave

FIGURE 2.1
CHANGES IN BODY WEIGHT AND COMPOSITION WITH AGE
FOR MALES AND FEMALES

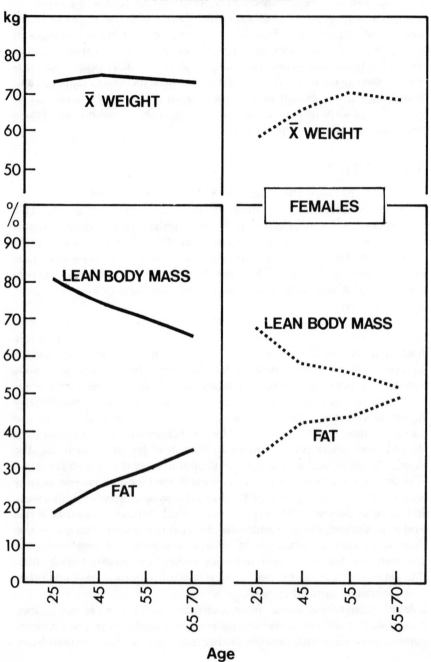

SOURCE: Forbes and Reina 1970

the circulatory system and, so, drug molecules bound to them are not free to leave the blood and cannot diffuse to their site of action. In effect, they are deactivated. For some drugs, as much as 99% of the molecules become protein bound, and for drugs like this, changes in the concentration of blood proteins and in their ability to bind drugs can considerably alter the amount of drug available at the site of action. Studies have shown that with age and some disease conditions, the concentration of blood proteins drops, and the binding ability of the remaining protein decreases (Greenblatt 1979). This means that those drugs that are normally highly bound to protein in young people will be less well bound in the aged. Consequently, there will be more drug available to get to the site of action in the elderly. Most tests of drug levels in the blood do not distinguish between bound and unbound drug and so similar blood levels may not mean similar concentration of the drug at the site of action in young and old individuals.

ELIMINATION

There are two main routes by which the body gets rid of unwanted substances. One route, metabolism, is controlled mainly by the liver and the other, excretion, is a function of the kidneys. The functioning of both organs normally changes as a result of age and, as a consequence, so does the body's ability to eliminate a drug.

The Kidneys

It is the function of the kidneys to remove substances from the blood and concentrate them in the urine for elimination. The functional unit of the kidney is the nephron, which is basically a long tube surrounded by a bed of fine blood vessels called capillaries. At one end of the nephron nearly all the fluid part of the blood is filtered into the tube. This fluid includes drugs and everything dissolved in the blood. As this filtered fluid passes through the nephron, the water and other substances the body needs are reabsorbed through the walls of the nephron into the blood in the capillaries that surround it. What is not reabsorbed is collected at the other end of the nephron in the urinary bladder and excreted from the body as urine. All substances reclaimed by the nephron must be reabsorbed through a membrane that forms the walls of the tube and, as in the digestive system, this means that drugs that have low lipid solubility or are ionized will be poorly reabsorbed and therefore excreted efficiently by the kidney. On the other hand, drugs that are highly lipid soluble will not be efficiently eliminated by the kidneys.

All functions of the kidneys have been shown to decline with age. The kidneys receive less blood from the heart (35% less in the elderly) (Greenblatt *et al.* 1982), the total size of the kidneys decreases and the number and functioning of nephrons decreases. Most of these changes take place after the fourth or fifth decade of life and result in higher blood levels and longer duration of action of drugs which depend on the kidneys for elimination (Mayersohn 1979).

The Liver

The second means the body uses to get rid of substances is metabolism, the process of changing the chemical structure of the drug molecules. This is primarily accomplished in the liver by means of enzymes. An enzyme is a catalyst of a chemical reaction, that is, its presence facilitates a chemical change, but it is not used up in that reaction and does not otherwise participate in the reaction. The type and speed of the chemical reactions that take place in the body are controlled by the amount and type of enzymes. For the most part, the result of these chemical changes is a molecule that is less physiologically active than the original drug molecule and one that is less lipid soluble or more easily ionized so the kidneys can excrete it more easily, but this is not always the case. The new substances created by metabolism, called metabolites, are sometimes more active than the parent drug. This is true for drugs like diazepam (Valium) that have a very long-lasting metabolite which seems to be responsible for much of the effect of the drug.

A useful scheme for discussing liver function is to describe the process of metabolism as having two phases. Phase 1 involves processes like oxidization, where relatively minor changes are made in the drug molecule. These changes have little effect on the activity of the drug, but make it slightly easier for it to be eliminated by the kidneys. In Phase 2, more complex changes take place that involve attaching the product of Phase 1 metabolism to another large molecule. The result is usually a substance that is without any physiological activity and is easily eliminated by the kidneys. Age appears to cause impairment of some types of Phase 1 metabolism, but there are few effects of age on Phase 2. This means for some drugs, the initial stages of metabolism will be slowed by age and this will cause the drug to build up to higher levels if it is taken repeatedly (Greenblatt *et al.* 1982).

The amount of enzyme available to metabolize a drug can be increased by a process known as induction. When some drugs are taken, enzyme systems in the liver are stimulated so that the next time that drug is administered there will be more enzyme available for its metabolism. The drug will have less effect after it is taken several times because it will be metabolized more quickly. Enzyme induction is not specific to one drug. Taking one drug can also induce the enzymes that metabolize a different drug. Cigarette smoking and heavy drinking, for example, will decrease the potency of many other drugs taken at the same time, like barbiturates and anesthetics, by inducing the enzymes that destroy them. There is some evidence that enzyme induction is reduced in older people (Mayersohn 1982). This could mean that the elderly might be slower to develop some types of tolerance to the effects of drugs, and alterations made in drug dose for smokers and drinkers may be inappropriate for the elderly.

Another age-related change that influences liver function is that blood flow to the liver decreases by about 40 to 45% between the ages of 20 and 65. Because it is the blood that brings the drug to the liver, this decrease reduces the exposure of the drug to enzymes and reduces metabolism. In addition, total liver size is reduced with age, and this would also be expected to reduce the efficiency of the liver (Greenblatt *et al.* 1982; Mayersohn 1982).

Illness and Disease

Most of the changes discussed so far are normal changes that occur with age, but older people are also likely to suffer from chronic diseases that can alter the functioning of many of the organs important in absorption, distribution and elimination. The effect of diseases of the liver, kidney and digestive system will be obvious, but other types of disease can also be important. For example, congestive heart failure can reduce absorption by decreasing blood flow to the intestine (Benet *et al.* 1976). Reduced blood flow to the liver and kidneys will also decrease the effectiveness of these organs (Mayersohn 1982).

Chronic illness that enforces bed rest can influence drug distribution because patterns of blood flow change in recumbent as opposed to ambulatory patients (Levy 1967). Indeed, decreases in physical activity brought on by ill health or changes in activity level will also alter patterns of blood distribution by altering blood flow to sites of drug absorption and action.

Chronic disease, poor nourishment and inactivity can decrease blood protein levels and the degree to which proteins can bind drugs. The result is that drugs that are normally protein bound will be more readily available at both their site of action and for metabolism and excretion (Greenblatt *et al.* 1982).

DRUG INTERACTIONS

Because the elderly have a greater tendency to take more drugs simultaneously than younger people (See Figure 3.3), they are more likely to experience adverse drug interactions. Drug interactions can take place at any stage of absorption, distribution, interaction with site of action, metabolism or excretion, and can take the form of either an increase or a decrease in the effect of a drug. The following are a few examples of pharmacokinetic interactions between drugs commonly taken by the elderly.

Because of frequent problems with digestion, the elderly often consume laxatives and antacids. Antacids decrease the acidity of the stomach and this can have the effect of slowing, or even stopping the disintegration and dissolution of tablets. In addition, lowered acidity also tends to increase ionization of drugs like aspirin that are weak acids and consequently decreases their absorption. Antacids also lower the ionization of weak bases like morphine, and subsequently increase their absorption. Laxatives can also decrease the absorption of many drugs because they coat the lining of the intestine.

Many drugs compete for binding sites on the blood protein. Drugs with high affinity for these sites can displace others with a lower affinity. Thus, if a high affinity drug is taken after a low affinity drug, it will displace the low affinity drug and cause a great increase in circulation of unbound drug. A drug like diazepam (Valium), for example, is 99% bound to protein, so even a small decrease of one or two percent in bound molecules brought about by a competing drug will double the available diazepam (Bressler 1982). As another example, the normal percent of unbound salicylate (drugs like aspirin or ASA) is about 30% in the blood of an older person taking no other drugs, but when two other drugs are also being taken at the same time, this unbound proportion increases to 50%. The result is an increase in the salicylate available to the site of action of 166% (Wallace *et al.* 1976). The decreased ability of the blood of the elderly to bind drugs makes older people more susceptible to this type of interaction.

Not only do antacid drugs alter the absorption of other drugs from the digestive system, they can also change the pH (acidity or alkalinity) of the urine and influence the lipid solubility of some drugs in the urine. Because lipid soluble drugs are reabsorbed into the blood through the nephron wall, increases in lipid solubility diminish the capacity of the kidney to excrete a drug, and decreases in lipid solubility speed excretion. Lowering the acidity of the urine will speed the excretion of acidic drugs like aspirin or phenylbutazone, and slow the excretion of basic drugs like morphine.

AGE-RELATED CHANGES IN DRUG SENSITIVITIES

Up to this point the only changes that have been discussed have involved changes in kinetics that cause an increase or a decrease in the concentration of drug delivered to the site of action, but there is some evidence that there may be age-related changes in the sensitivity of receptors at the site of action of some drugs, or changes in the ability of these receptors to alter body physiology. Most drugs are believed to produce their effect by interacting with specific receptor sites in the body. These receptor sites are located on large protein molecules on the surface of body cells. When the drug molecule of the correct configuration is available, it will bind to the receptor, and this process causes a physiological change in the tissue where the receptor is located. It is not easy to determine whether an age-related change in the effect of a drug is the result of a change in the number of drug molecules at the receptor site (due to altered pharmacokinetics), or a change in the sensitivity of the drug receptor. However, there is evidence that some drugs, like benzodiazepines (diazepam and nitrazepam) and some anticoagulants may have a greater effect on older people, even at the same drug concentrations. This suggests that either there are more drug receptors in older people, or that the receptors for these drugs are more sensitive. Elderly people may also have a reduced sensitivity to beta-adrenergic agonists and antagonists, drugs that are often taken for heart conditions.

CONCLUSIONS

While it can easily be demonstrated that there are many age-related changes in the body that can affect the pharmacokinetics of drugs, and that the sensitivity of the body to different drugs changes with age, the exact clinical significance of these findings has yet to be established and should be the subject of extended investigation. For example, we have seen that there are numerous studies that demonstrate age-related changes in the digestive system which might be expected to alter the absorption of many drugs, but a number of studies of actual absorption have failed to show any real age-related changes. On the other hand, age-related changes in metabolism appear to have considerable effect on the action of many drugs.

Two rather general conclusions can be made at this time. First, for most drugs, on the average, there is an increase in sensitivity with increasing age. Second, it is possible to conclude that the older the population, the more variability there will be in the response to drugs. While the older person will, on the average, be more sensitive to most drugs, it is very difficult to predict appropriate doses for any individual. Clearly there is a great need to know the individual factors apart from age that may predict how a particular individual of advanced age will respond to a specific drug. When such factors are determined, this knowledge should be widely distributed, not only to physicians, but to users of non-prescription drugs as well, perhaps on bottle labels or package inserts.

CHAPTER 3

PRESCRIPTION AND OVER-THE-COUNTER DRUGS

EXTENT OF DRUG USE

Introduction

From July 1978 to March 1979 Health and Welfare Canada and Statistics Canada undertook a survey of the health of Canadians in which they interviewed a randomly selected sample of 12,000 households (Canada Health Survey 1981). Among the many questions they asked were questions concerning medicines and drugs that individuals had taken in the last two days. The medicines they asked about included prescription drugs and over-the-counter (OTC) non-prescription drugs taken either with or without the advice of a physician. When these data are examined by age, some interesting patterns emerge. It is quite clear from Figure 3.1 that, as age increases, the use of most medications, both OTC and prescribed, increases. Many drugs, like those taken for high blood pressure, are used almost exclusively by those over 45. The one interesting exception to this trend is the use of antibiotics, which is higher in children, but decreases in adults and remains constant throughout the life span. All types of drugs, with the exception of antibiotics and stomach medicines, are used more by women than by men.

While most studies clearly show that drug use increases with age, it is difficult to identify exactly which drugs are the most widely used by the elderly because of variations in survey techniques, sample populations and definitions of drug categories. It also seems likely that different drugs are used by different populations in different parts of the country. Table 3.1 summarizes the relative frequency of use of several categories of drugs reported in four roughly comparable surveys of elderly populations. Three of these were conducted in Canada (Skelton 1985; Murray 1974; Canada Health Survey 1981), and one is from the United States (Guttman 1978). The most widely used drugs among all these populations are drugs that control cardiac and vascular disease. These account for 15 to 34% of all drugs reported. Tranquilizers and sleeping pills (barbiturates and benzodiazepines) account for 3 to 15% and analgesics and anti-inflammatory drugs

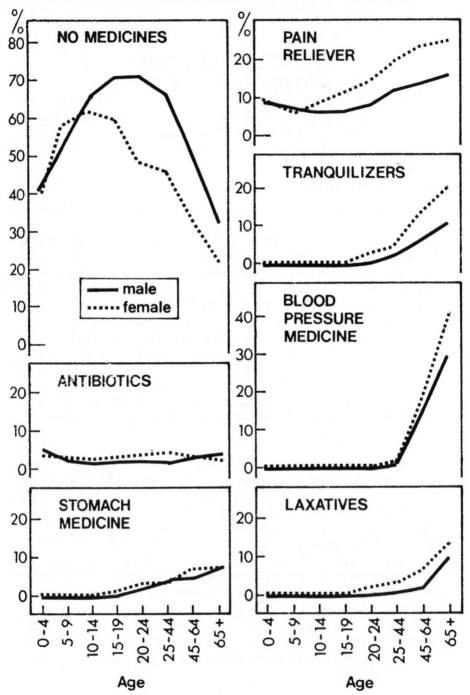

FIGURE 3.1

THE FREQUENCY OF THE USE OF VARIOUS TYPES OF PRESCRIPTION AND OTC MEDICINES IN CANADA BY SEX IN DIFFERENT AGE GROUPS

SOURCE: Canada Health Survey 1981, Table 95, p. 179.

vary from 9 to 20%. The notable feature about these data is the great variability between studies. For example, vitamins account for over 27% of all drugs reported by respondents in Skelton's (1985) survey in Edmonton, but less than 3% of the drugs in the Guttman (1978) survey in the United States. Laxatives vary from less than 1% to more than 11%.

Virtually all studies of drug use report that older people tend to take many medicines simultaneously, and that this trend increases with age. Figure 3.2 shows that in the Canada Health Survey, 13% of men and 25% of women over the age of 65 take three or more different drugs concurrently, whereas 4.2% of men and 8.9% of women in the entire sample take more than three drugs concurrently. A similar and more recent survey conducted by the American Association of Retired Persons (AARP) (1984) has shown that in the United States, there is a similar age-related tendency to use multiple medicines. The AARP survey found that 24% of those over 65 take more than three prescription drugs a day, compared with only 9% in the 45 to 64 age range.

TABLE 3.1

TYPES OF DRUGS USED BY ELDERLY REPORTED IN SEVERAL DIFFERENT SURVEYS IN CANADA AND THE UNITED STATES (PERCENT)

Drug Class	Skelton (1985)(1)	Murray (1974)(2)	NIDA (1977)(3)	Canada Health Survey (1981)(4)
cardioactive vasoactive and diuretics	21.7	15.0	20.3	34.4
tranquilizers and hypnotics	8.5	8.8	2.8	15.6
vitamins	27.6	7.9	2.8	5.3
analgesic and anti-inflammatory	15.8	9.5	11.8	20.9
laxatives	5.2	11.1	0.9	11.0
total drugs	492	559	1075	2019

SOURCES: (1) Skelton (1985) — members of seniors association in Edmonton, all "relatively healthy" and non-institutionalized, 50+ years — drugs consumed daily
(2) Murray (1974) — non-selected sample from Winnipeg, 32% in institutions, 60+ years — drugs consumed in the last three days
(3) NIDA (Guttman 1978) — stratified sample of non-institutionalized elderly from census tracts of Washington D.C., 60+ years — drugs used daily
(4) Canada Health Survey (1981) — random sample of non-institutionalized Canadians, 60+ — drugs consumed in the past two days.

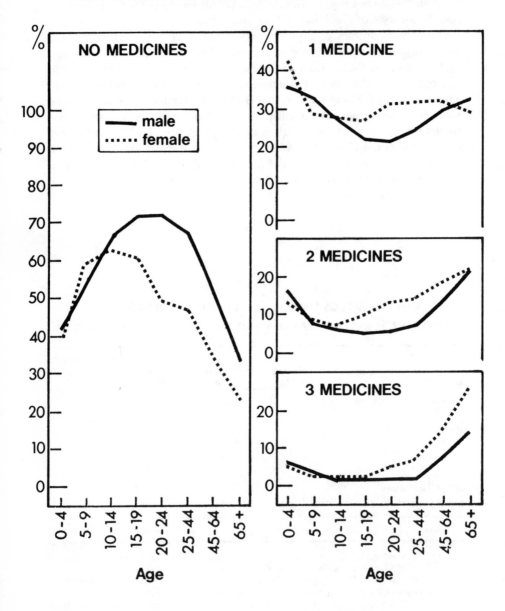

FIGURE 3.2

TOTAL NUMBER OF DIFFERENT PRESCRIBED AND OTC MEDICINES TAKEN BY CANADIANS IN THE TWO DAYS PRIOR TO THE SURVEY

SOURCE: Canada Health Survey 1981, Table 96, p. 180.

VARIABLES RELATED TO INCREASED DRUG USE

Disease and Perceived Health

There are several possible explanations for this increase in drug use with age. The most obvious is that the elderly tend to have more chronic illness and can benefit from drug therapy. (Older persons have fewer acute illnesses such as viral infections [Mishara and Riedel 1984], but acute illnesses tend to last longer in the elderly.) In the Canada Health Survey, those over 65 accounted for 20.4% of those reporting health problems, while this age group accounts for only 8.8% of the population sample. The elderly were similarly over-represented in nearly every category of health problems except for influenza and acute respiratory difficulties such as hay fever. Clearly, older people have more chronic disease, and this is responsible for much of the increase in medicine use seen with age. In one study in the United States, Guttman (1978) reported a significant positive correlation between the use of medicines (both prescription and OTC) and poor health and physical disability. He also reported that nearly 40% of the elderly population that he sampled claimed that they would be unable to carry on their daily activities all or part of the time without their prescription drugs. A further 8% reported being similarly dependent on OTC drugs. Alcohol use was negatively correlated with reported poor health and disabilities, and with the use of medicines.

If poor health is a major contributor to the use of drugs by older people, it would follow that for those who have no health problems there should be no increase in drug use with age. The study by Skelton (1985) provides partial support for this prediction. In the Skelton survey, a sample of 245 persons who were members of the Edmonton Society for the Retired and Semi-Retired were asked about their medical history and about the details of any pharmacological agents that they were taking. The age of the respondents ranged from 50 to 88, and all participants considered themselves "relatively healthy." While it was found that women took more than twice the number of drugs as men, there was no increase in the number of drugs taken as age increased. This suggests that for a healthy population, age does not inevitably indicate an increased use of drugs. It should be noted, however, that the average number of medicines used regularly by this "fit" population was 2.0, and one respondent took 11 drugs regularly.

Clearly, health status is a major predictor of the use of medicines by older people, but it is far from being the only factor. In a recent study by McKim, Stones and Kozma (1986) 401 people over the age of 65 in Newfoundland were interviewed on two occasions 18 months apart. A regression analysis was performed relating their use of medicines to a wide variety of other social, psychological and demographic variables. It was found that the best predictor of drug use was the presence of disease and its severity, but closely following actual disease was a self-rating of general health on a seven-point scale. Since the statistical analysis accounted for the effect of reported disease and severity, this measure reflected perceived health problems rather than real health problems. This suggests that thinking you are unhealthy is almost as important a factor in determining drug use as being unhealthy.

Another related area that requires attention from researchers is the role played by physicians in providing these drugs. If perceived ill health, as opposed to actual ill health, is a cause of increased prescription drug use, then physicians are not doing their job. As we shall see, most of the problems caused by drugs in older people are a result of taking many drugs at the same time. Clearly, physicians should only be prescribing drugs for "real" rather than "perceived" ill health in order to reduce the problems caused by taking too many medicines at once.

Physician Prescribing Practices

It is possible that increased use of medicines is partly due to greater exposure to physicians that arises from diminished health. In the Canada Health Survey, 20% (410/2019) of those over 65 reported visiting a physician 10 or more times a year, while the population average is 9.4%. There are those who speculate that physicians tend to respond to all complaints with a "technical solution," meaning a drug prescription, whether the patient really requires medication or not (Waldron 1977; Mandolini 1981). This problem is no doubt exacerbated by the influence of advertising in medical journals by drug companies (Butler 1975). It might follow, then, that the elderly, who see physicians more often than younger people, would be exposed to more "technical solutions." Data collected by the American Association of Retired Persons survey suggest that physicians do indeed rely almost exclusively on such technical solutions. Seventy-three percent of those over 65 report that their physician never suggests any other solution for their problem than taking the drug being prescribed. This reliance on drugs, however, is not limited to the treatment of older people, since 68% of all those surveyed reported the same lack of alternative treatment suggestions (AARP 1984).

It has been suggested that there is a built-in bias among physicians to devalue the final years of life. Some physicians appear to feel that it is more important to relieve the stresses of health problems with psychoactive drugs like Valium rather than to become involved in more time-consuming rehabilitation (Mock 1977; Mandolini 1981). Indeed, the increased use of tranquilizers among the elderly seems to suggest that this may be the case. A survey of the use and attitudes of physicians towards minor tranquilizers (Chambers *et al.* 1983) is related to this issue. The survey was conducted on a sample of members of the Texas Medical Association and found that 20% of all prescriptions for minor tranquilizers were being written for people over the age of 60. It was also found that physicians who were likely to prescribe these drugs often, and for long periods of time, were more likely to (a) be general practitioners, (b) be in a solo practice rather than a group practice, (c) carry a larger patient load, and (d) be out of medical school for a long time. These physicians also reported less training and experience in handling problems related to anxiety and less general knowledge about pharmacology. (Several mistakenly identified antidepressants and anti-psychotics as minor tranquilizers.) It is not known whether older people are more likely to see physicians in solo practice or with a large patient load, but it is more than likely that family physicians of older people are themselves older, and consequently, they are likely to have been out of medical school for a long time. This would mean that they would have less knowl-edge of pharmacology and be more likely to prescribe (and mis-prescribe) tranquilizers. Given the rapid expansion of drugs now available to the modern physician, it is not surprising that many physicians do not fully understand the actions of the drugs they prescribe. It has been pointed out that half of today's physicians were in medical school when 70% of all drugs now available were unknown or not available (Olson and Johnson 1977).

In a report of the Royal College of Physicians of London (1984) excessive prescribing was identified as one of the major causes of adverse drug reac-tions in the elderly. This report suggested that doctors often over-prescribe because of pressure from both the patient and pharmaceutical manufac-turer. They also suggest that pharmacological treatment offered by physi-cians may be "enthusiastic," "over-energetic" and "inappropriate."

While it is likely that physicians play a role in the increased medication of the elderly, they are clearly not solely responsible. An examination of the types of drugs taken by the elderly shows that the drugs they use are not ones exclusively prescribed by a physician. An American survey (May *et al.* 1982) has shown that over 28% of all drugs taken by a sample of elderly people were not prescribed by a physician. Similarly, a survey by Murray (1974) of a sample of elderly people in Winnipeg showed that 42% of the drugs taken were OTC drugs, representing an average of 2.4 drugs per per-son. In addition, drugs like laxatives that are widely used by the elderly are not frequently given on prescription. In fact, only 50% of those taking laxa-tives in the Canada Health Survey took them on the advice of a physician. Antibiotics, on the other hand, are not a class of drugs overused by the aged, and they are available only on prescription. Quite clearly, older people themselves are responsible for much of the age-related increase in the use of medicines.

Sex Differences

In most developed countries, it is widely reported that at all ages, the death rate for males is higher than for females. However, all measures of the use of health care services, including the use of medicines, show that females have higher rates than males. This sex difference varies with age. It is most marked in the 25 to 44 age group where the ratio of women to men taking more than three different drugs is 3.22 to 1. In the over 65 group this ratio is reduced to 1.9 to 1 (Canada Health Survey 1981). While some of the differences between the sexes are due to reproductive factors during childbearing years, they cannot entirely be accounted for by such biological differences. It is widely believed that social and cultural factors are even more important determinants of sex differences in health care-related behaviours, including medicine taking (Whittington *et al.* 1981; Nathanson 1975, 1977). There are those who argue that the nurturant roles of women in our society prevent women from taking good care of themselves and, consequently, they suffer more than men from mental illness and mild physical illness. These disorders require more attention from physicians and more drug treatment, but are not life-threatening and do not increase the mortality rates of women, which are consistently lower than for men (Grove and Hughes 1979). Others suggest that there are sex role-related differences in defining and reporting illness (Marcus and Seeman 1981). The debate over these issues is fascinating, extensive, complex and beyond the scope of this book. For a more complete discussion, the reader is referred to the previous references as well as Phillips and Segal (1969).

Since many of these drugs are prescribed by a physician, it is possible that this sex difference represents sex-related differences in prescribing practices. Physicians may be more likely to prescribe drugs to women than to men. Women go to doctors more often than men, and the age-related pattern of visits to doctors resembles the age-related drug-use changes. Doctor visits are higher during childhood and then drop off to a low level in the 20 to 45 age group, after which they increase with age. Throughout adult life, women consult doctors more frequently than men, although, like multiple drug use, this sex difference diminishes with age. Statistics Canada (1984) has reported that among those over 65, 17.7% of men and 22.4% women have more than 10 consultations with a physician in a year, whereas in the total Canadian population 6.7% of men and 12.1% of women make more than 10 visits a year to a physician. If the increased use of medications in the elderly and in women is solely a result of the prescribing practices of physicians, we might expect that it would be apparent only for prescription drugs, which is not the case in the Canada Health Survey. In a survey of the general population in the United States, 70% of women as opposed to 58% of men took non-prescription drugs (May *et al.* 1982). Clearly, age-related as well as sex-related increases in medicine use can not be entirely a result of biases in physician prescribing practices.

Stress, Life Satisfaction and Other Variables

One view holds that the elderly take more drugs as a response to the stresses associated with aging. This might well be an explanation for the increased use by the elderly of psychotropic drugs such as the benzodiazepines. One survey in the United States showed that prescription drug use was not only correlated with ill health, but high medication users tended to be less satisfied with their lives and had a lower perception of themselves in terms of intelligence and capacity. Psychotropic drug use was also correlated with family relationships that were perceived as unsatisfactory, and with lower levels of life satisfaction (Guttman 1978). Eve and Friedsam (1981) studied tranquilizer and sleeping pill use in a population of older people in Texas. They found that the use of these drugs was related not only to general health, but also to other variables such as loneliness and dissatisfaction with income.

While these studies seem to indicate that satisfaction and life events are contributing factors, more recent Canadian data suggest that this may not be so. In the study by McKim *et al.* (1986) reported above, it was shown that disease and perceived health contributed significantly to medicine use. Other factors like locus of control and word fluency were also significant predictors of drug use, but variables like age, sex, satisfaction with finances and housing and happiness were not significant predictors. Clearly more of this type of research investigating many variables at the same time is needed in order to achieve a more adequate understanding of the factors that seem to cause drug use.

If increased drug use were a response to increased stress brought about by aging and dissatisfaction, we might expect that there would be an increase in the use of recreational drugs like alcohol, tobacco and caffeine. Not only does the use of all these recreational drugs decline with age, but it has also been shown that users of prescription and OTC medicines are more likely to abstain from alcohol (Guttman 1978). In addition, if drug use in the elderly is fulfilling a psychological rather than a medical function, it might be expected that older people would take their prescription drugs more frequently than they were supposed to, and like other age groups that abuse prescription drugs, they would resort to such subterfuges as visiting several different physicians in order to obtain increased amounts of the drug. The following section on compliance shows this is not the case. Older people are much more likely to underuse than overuse prescribed drugs. While there are reports that some old people acquire multiple prescriptions for psychoactive drugs and deliberately over-medicate themselves (Glantz 1981; Pascarelli and Fischer 1974), the extent to which these practices occur and their relationship to age have not been adequately assessed. Deliberate self-medication of psychotropic drugs like tranquilizers does not, however, appear to be a major problem in elderly populations.

Institutionalization

The population sampled by the Canada Health Survey excluded people living in institutions. For those interested in drug use in other populations, this is a significant omission. This population appears to take even more drugs than the non-institutionalized elderly. A study conducted in the United States has shown that expenditures on non-psychotropic drugs by the institutionalized are only slightly greater than in the non-institutionalized elderly, but those in institutions spend 17 times more on psychotropic drugs (Glazer and Zawadski 1981). This study showed that 40% of all drugs prescribed to the elderly in institutions were psychotropic drugs. Moreover, the psychotropic drugs favoured were not necessarily the benzodiazepine tranquilizers used by the non-institutionalized elderly, but were more usually stronger drugs (Zawadski *et al.* 1978). While there are reports of over-medication of the institutionalized elderly in Canada (Mallett and Gervais 1984), the extent and nature of medication use associated with institutionalization have not been adequately studied in Canada. There is, however, no reason to believe that the pattern in Canada is different from that in the United States.

While it is to be expected that people in institutions will be in need of increased medicines due to illness, there is not an increase in psychiatric disorders in the elderly that can account for this vast increase in psychiatric drugs. It has been suggested by Butler (1975) that much of the use of psychotropic drugs for the elderly, including antipsychotics, is motivated by a desire to control the person rather than to treat and improve symptoms. Butler uses the term "pacification" to suggest that in institutions the pacifying action of antipsychotics and antidepressants "... makes them tempting substitutes for decent, humane attention through diagnosis and careful treatment." (Butler 1975).

COMPLIANCE IN THE ELDERLY

> If we look dispassionately at both sides of the "compliance-prescribance" axis some sort of rough-and-ready natural law seems to be at work, balancing the interests of both physician and patient: The physician will be expected to prescribe with only approximate accuracy, and the patient will be expected to comply with only modest fidelity. Thus mankind has been able to survive bleeding, cupping, leaches, mustard plasters, turpentine stupes and Panalba. (Charney 1975).

The term "compliance" (some prefer "adherence") refers to the degree to which a patient conforms (or adheres) to, or complies with, the instructions of a physician. While "compliance" may well include keeping appointments and maintaining a special diet, here we will be talking about how well people follow instructions about taking medicines. There are several different types of non-compliance which include under-compliance — not taking as much as prescribed, over-compliance — taking more than prescribed or taking a drug that was not prescribed, and schedule non-compliance — taking the right medicine, but at the wrong time (Hulka 1979). Some researchers also include a lack of knowledge or understanding of the purpose or actions of a drug as a type of non-compliance (Schwartz *et al.* 1962).

Age and Compliance with Drug Regimens

There are many reasons to believe that older people may be non-compliant. It has been reported frequently that the elderly have a hard time getting the top off child-proof medicine bottles (Atkinson *et al.* 1978) and because of impaired vision, may have difficulty reading the labels on bottles or be unable to identify pills accurately (Hurd *et al.* 1984). In addition, the elderly may also be forgetful or have difficulty understanding the instructions of a physician because of hearing problems.

Surveys have shown a very high rate of non-compliance in older people. In an early study, Schwartz *et al.* (1962) studied the compliance of 178 ambulatory patients over 60 years old who had at least one diagnosed chronic disease and were taking at least one medicine. This study considered lack of understanding of the purpose of the medicines as an error. They found that 59% made some sort of medication error (many made more than one) and 26% made an error that was potentially serious. Sixty-four percent of patients made errors of omission. About 41% were confused and did not understand the nature of the drugs they had been given, 36% took other medicines that had been prescribed at other times or to other people. There were also frequent errors in scheduling and dosage. Other studies have also found a variety of compliance rates in older populations. These studies are difficult to compare because of different techniques for assessing compliance and different definitions of compliance. There is also reason to believe that different survey techniques are not equally accurate in assessing compliance. This problem is further discussed in Chapter 6.

Law and Chalmers (1976) reported a compliance rate of 75%, with the majority of errors being errors of omission. Cooper *et al.* (1984) surveyed people over 60 years old and found 57% compliant, with 90% of errors being drug omission. A study by Kiernan and Isaacs (1981) surveyed 50 patients over the age of 65. They found that 65% of the medicines (both prescription and OTC) were being taken at the correct dose and 30% were being taken at less than the prescribed dose. Only 6% were being taken in doses larger than recommended. In a study by Stephens *et al.* (1981) of the use of psychoactive drugs by those over 55, it was found that only 7% reported that they did not always follow the prescription directions, and 87% of those took the drug less often than prescribed.

In a survey of 236 clinic patients over 60, Neely and Patric (1968) found that 59% were making no errors, and half of the errors made were omission. MacDonald *et al.* (1977) surveyed 165 elderly patients after discharge from Sherwood Hospital in Britain. They found an overall compliance rate of 54% after one week, and a 38% compliance rate at 12 weeks. Errors of omission represented 75% of errors at one week and 65% at 12 weeks after discharge.

While it seems quite clear that older people make many errors in drug use, are they more likely to make mistakes than any other segment of the population? In the above studies, the compliance rates ranged from 38% to 93% in older people. This does not appear to be any different than the compliance rate for the general population. In a study of patients not selected by age, Ettlinger and Freeman (1981) found 50% compliance after four or five days in 119 patients prescribed an antibiotic. Parkin *et al.* (1976) found a 74.1% compliance rate in a group of patients 10 days after they were discharged from hospital. In a review of studies, Stewart and Cluff (1972) reported that compliance rates ranged from 41% to 75%, roughly the same range found in studies of the elderly.

A number of other studies have directly examined the effect of age on compliance and, with some exceptions, these studies also suggest that age is not related to compliance, or if it is, the relationship is complex and not understood. In the study by Schwartz *et al.* (1962), they found that error rates for drug taking were slightly higher in those over 75 than in those aged 60 to 75, but a more precise breakdown of errors by age showed no consistent change. In fact, the highest compliance rate, 70% was seen in patients over 80, the oldest age group. In a study of 190 patients discharged consecutively from Victoria General Hospital in Halifax, Brand *et al.* (1977) found no statistically significant effect of age on compliance. They did find that compliance decreased steadily from 74% in the 40 to 49 age group to 27.5% in the over 80 group, but the second highest non-compliance rate (50%) was in the 30 to 39 age group. Other studies have looked at age and have not found significant effects (Neely and Patric 1968; Parkin *et al.* 1976; Ettlinger and Freeman 1981; German *et al.* 1984; Cooper *et al.* 1984; Stephens *et al.* 1981).

One study found that older people were actually better compliers than middle-aged people. A survey conducted by the American Association of Retired Persons (AARP 1984) asked respondents whether they had ever failed to have a prescription filled or whether they had ever discontinued taking a drug prescribed by their doctor after they started to use it. The survey showed that 86% of older Americans always filled prescriptions and, once filled, 67% never discontinued using them. In contrast, middle-aged Americans (aged 45-65) only filled prescriptions 74% of the time, and 57% always followed the full course of medication. Elderly Americans did better than the middle-aged group on other compliance measures as well. Only 9% of older people admitted to either borrowing someone else's medicine or lending theirs to someone else, while 17% of the middle-aged group engaged in the practice.

In all age groups, by far the most common type of non-compliance reported is under-compliance or drug defaulting. In older people, it has been suggested that under-compliance may be a result of a number of age-related factors such as confusion or lack of understanding of the drug regimen (Schwartz et al. 1962; Das 1977), inability to open childproof containers, inability to read instructions in small type (Atkinson et al. 1977, 1978), or the expense of the drug (Brand et al. 1977). Indeed, many studies have shown that these factors contribute to under-compliance, but most research shows that the majority of under-compliance in all age groups is deliberate. In addition to the AARP survey just discussed, one study by Cooper et al. (1984) found that 73% of under-compliance in an elderly population was intentional. In this study, the reasons given for under-compliance are interesting. Fifty-two percent of intentional under-users said that they did not take the drug because they did not think that they needed it. Only 15% said that they cut down or stopped the drug because of side effects. In the AARP survey, older people were asked why they failed to have prescriptions filled. Fifty-one percent said that they thought the drug would not help, or that their condition improved and they did not need it. Thirty percent expressed concern about side effects. Among those that discontinue a prescription drug after they have started to use it, the figures are reversed; 55% were concerned about side effects and 25% stopped the drug because their condition improved and they did not think they needed it. Twenty-five percent stopped their drug because they did not think it was helping.

Another interesting finding of the AARP survey is that 52% of those who did not fill a prescription, and 34% of those who stopped taking a prescribed drug did not tell their physician. This reluctance to tell physicians that their advice is being ignored is understandable, but it does indicate a serious lack of communication between physician and patient. We have already noted that physicians generally do not tell their patients what they might do for their problem apart from taking a drug. Later in this chapter we will show that communication between physician and patient is an important determinant of drug compliance.

The study by Brand et al. (1977) of patients discharged from Victoria General Hospital in Halifax found a different reason for under-compliance — cost. Thirty-six percent failed to comply because of the cost of the drug. Cost of drugs was a factor for only 6% of the respondents in the AARP survey. The difference may well be that the AARP survey was based on a random sample of the entire elderly population while the Brand study was based on those discharged from hospital. This latter population might be expected to be in poorer health, be taking many more medicines and incurring greater cost. In fact, the Brand study does show that non-compliance was greater in those that were carrying a vary costly prescription load. The average cost of drugs for those who did not comply was three times greater than for those who did comply.

Stephens et al. (1981) asked elderly defaulters of prescription psychoactive drugs why they took less of the drug than prescribed. Almost half (48.6%) said simply that they did not like the medicine. Twenty-three percent said that they only took a drug when they felt that they needed it. Fewer than 10% said that cost was a factor.

We have already examined the effect of age on compliance and determined that there does not appear to be a systematic effect of aging on compliance, but are there any other identifiable factors that do affect compliance? In a review of patient characteristics, Hulka (1979) determined that the following characteristics are not related to compliance: age, sex, marital status, education, current activity, number of people in the household and social class. In addition, the type of medication and the specific diagnosis also have little effect (Haynes 1976). Most of the literature on compliance in the aging supports these conclusions. While the personal characteristics of the patient have little influence, it has been clearly demonstrated that there are factors that do alter compliance. These are related to the complexity of the treatment and the degree of understanding and comprehension of the patient.

Treatment Characteristics

Two reviews of the literature on characteristics of the treatment regimen and compliance by Blackwell (1979) and Haynes *et al.* (1977), show that the frequency with which a drug must be taken does not seem to have any great effect on compliance. However, these reviews do show that there is clear agreement among studies that the number of different drugs prescribed at any one time has a clear effect on compliance; compliance falls off sharply when the number of different medications reaches three or more a day. Studies of elderly drug-takers confirm that compliance deteriorates sharply as number of prescriptions increases (Neely and Patric 1968; Parkin *et al.* 1976), but with the elderly, the frequency of dose was also important in some studies (Parkin *et al.* 1976; German *et al.* 1984), but not in others (Kiernan and Isaacs 1981). Since it has been shown that older people are much more likely than young people to be taking more than three drugs at any one time, we might expect that compliance could be much more difficult for them to maintain.

Understanding and Communication

Another factor that influences compliance is understanding. Patients who are able to identify all the drugs they are taking and describe both the medical condition for which the medicine was prescribed and the prescription schedule generally seem to make fewer errors than those who cannot. In a study by Hulka (1979), a number of doctor-patient pairs were studied, and it was demonstrated that patients who were able to identify the function of all their drugs made fewer errors of commission and fewer scheduling errors than patients who could not. Not surprisingly, it was also shown that the ability to identify drug function decreased as the number of prescribed drugs increased. Another study by German *et al.* (1984) compared patients above and below 65 years of age on their knowledge of their diseases and medications. In general, those over 65 knew less about their illnesses and drugs than those under 65, and for both groups the ability to identify drugs correctly diminished greatly as the number of prescriptions increased. They found that greater knowledge was associated with greater compliance, but the effect was not statistically significant.

We have already noted that physicians do not always explain alternatives to drugs to their patients and patients do not always tell their doctor when they do not take a prescribed drug. This lack of communication can affect compliance. Both the Hulka and the German *et al.* studies examined the degree of communication between the patient and the physician. In the German *et al.* study it was shown that there was a consistent positive relationship between perceived communication with the physician and correct knowledge and compliance at all ages. Hulka questioned physicians on what they had told their patients about their disease, and patients were asked what they knew about their disease. By comparing these two sources of information it was possible to generate a communication score for each doctor-patient pair. The degree of communication was related to all types of compliance, the better the communication, the better the compliance. The role of the physician-patient relationship has been shown to be important in many other compliance studies (Atkinson *et al.* 1977; Smith and Andrews 1983; Ettinger and Freeman 1981) and improved understanding and communication have been shown to improve compliance in an elderly population (Wandless and Davie 1977).

ADVERSE REACTIONS TO MEDICINES

On many occasions, medicines have effects that are not wanted. These effects may or may not be serious, but they are referred to as Drug Adverse Reactions (DAR) or Medicine Adverse Reactions.[1] What constitutes a Drug Adverse Reaction? This question has been answered in various ways at various times, and the diversity of definitions makes it difficult to understand how the published research on DAR's relates to aging. One of the best definitions, and the one we will be adopting, defines a DAR as any effect of a drug not wanted by either the physician or the patient. This definition does not distinguish between DAR's and side effects, and we will be using the terms interchangeably. A side effect is an effect that occurs along with the main or therapeutic effect of a drug and is not normally considered (at least by the physician) to be serious. A dry mouth or sleepiness may be considered to be side effects. Some of the research reported below would not include these side effects as DAR's, but other studies do. It is not always apparent what definition a particular study is using, but where possible, we have indicated which definition is being used.

There have been a number of different surveys that have attempted to relate the frequency of Drug Adverse Reactions to age. The conclusions reached by these studies depend upon such things as whether the survey includes illicit drugs, the population surveyed and whether the definition of DAR includes addiction and deliberate or accidental overdose. Two large American surveys seem to show that older people are under-represented among those showing DAR's. The Drug Abuse Warning Network (DAWN) (DHEW U.S. 1979) is a United States nationwide system that monitors drug abuse contacts from hospital admissions, emergency rooms, crisis centres and medical examiners (coroners). In the years 1974–1975, DAWN reported that only 5% of its contacts were with people over the age of 50 even though this group represents 26% of the U.S. population. The reason for this under-representation is probably because DAWN monitors events that include illegal drugs of abuse such as marijuana, heroin and hallucinogens. This would tend to increase the representation of younger people and decrease the percent of the elderly, who, as we shall see in Chapter 5, do not use these drugs to any extent, or at least did not in the middle 1970s. The DAWN data show that even for DAR's caused by many prescription drugs, people over 50 are under-represented. For example, of all the cases reported involving pentobarbital, only 16% were for those over 50. DAR's caused by other barbiturates and benzodiazepines were reported with even less frequency for the elderly.

In another large-scale study, the emergency room records for Miami's Jackson Memorial Hospital during the period of January 1, 1972 to June 30, 1976, were examined for reports of primary complaints that involved drugs (excluding alcohol, but included overdoses and suicides). Only 2.6% of these cases involved people over 60. This age group represents 10% of the population of the catchment area for that hospital (Inciardi *et al.* 1978). In the Jackson Memorial study, 21.8% of all drugs reported were illicit, but there were no reports of anyone over 60 having a DAR from an illicit drug. Those over 60, however, reported the highest frequency of problems with OTC medications (8% of admissions over 60 years old) and some prescription drugs (17%).

Studies of hospital admissions for drug reactions that exclude suicide and addiction or drug abuse tell a completely different story. Caranasos *et al.* (1974) studied admissions to the University of Florida Teaching Hospital for a three-year period. Of 6,063 admissions, 2.9% were due to drug-induced illness. People over 60 accounted for 31.5% of all hospital admissions for all causes for that period, but constituted 41.2% of DAR admissions. Women were also over-represented. In a similar study by Hurwitz (1969) in Belfast, of those over 60 admitted to hospital, 15.4% were admitted for a DAR to medication, compared with 6.3% of those under 60.

Health and Welfare Canada keeps extensive records of DAR's reported by hospitals and physicians across Canada. The Health and Welfare Canada figures represent unwanted drug effects that have occurred at recommended therapeutic doses and do not include suicides or accidental overdose. Table 3.2 shows the total number of reported DAR's by sex and age for the years 1980 to 1984. Reports for which age and sex were not reported accounted for 7.5% of the total and have been omitted from this table. Table 3.2 also gives the population of Canada in each of these age and sex categories. These two distributions were compared using a Chi-square test[2] which showed that people over 65 are reported to have DAR's with a frequency greater than that which would be expected by chance (Chi-square = 7489.89, df = 1, p < .001).[3]

Seidl and his associates (Seidl *et al.* 1966) studied the incidence of DAR's among inpatients of Johns Hopkins Hospital. In four wards of patients with various acute medical conditions, they found that patients over 50 experienced DAR's at a rate of 17.4%. For those under 60 the rate was 11.9%. Patients between 51 and 60 had a mean DAR rate of 14.3%, those 61 to 70 had a rate of 15.7%, 71 to 80 had a rate of 18.3% and patients over 80 had a rate of 24%. Females also had a higher rate than males (8% for males as compared with 19.2% for females). In this study, a DAR was defined as any response to a drug that was unintended and undesired by the physician who prescribed it.

While it seems apparent that DAR's are more common in the elderly, it is still not clear why. There is certainly reason to believe that altered pharmacokinetics and increased sensitivity to drugs will lead to increased DAR's, but is this the only reason that older people are over-represented in these surveys? There is good evidence that many of these DAR's arise from the increased number of drugs taken by older people.

TABLE 3.2

PERCENT DISTRIBUTION OF REPORTED DAR'S IN CANADA FROM 1980 TO 1984 BY AGE AND SEX/EXPECTED FREQUENCY BASED UPON POPULATION STATISTICS

sex	age		
	less than 65	65+	total
male	28.80/46.01	10.96/3.78	39.76/49.79
female	43.54/45.34	16.70/4.43	60.24/50.21
total	72.34/91.35	27.66/8.68	100.0/100.0
Chi-square = 7489, df = 1, p < .01			

SOURCE: Health and Welfare Canada.

In a survey of patients admitted to geriatric medicine departments in England, Wales and Scotland, 15.3% showed DAR's (Williamson and Chopin 1980). These researchers also found that there was no difference between those under and over 75 in the frequency of DAR's, but one factor that contributed greatly to the probability of a DAR was the number of prescription drugs that person was taking. Patients taking one drug had a rate of 10.8%, while those taking six had a rate of 27%. In another study of hospitalized patients by Hurwitz, she found that those receiving fewer than five drugs accounted for 19% of all DAR's, while those who received more than six drugs accounted for 81% of all reported DAR's (Hurwitz 1969).

May *et al.* (1977) have also shown that the incidence of DAR's is related to the number of drugs used. They studied over 10,000 hospitalized patients for a five-year period and found that the probability of experiencing a DAR to any category of drug increased as the number of drugs concurrently taken increased. While the May *et al.* study did not report on the effects of age of the patient, the findings are of particular interest because the categories of drugs that caused by far the greatest incidence of DAR's were antihypertensives and anticoagulants, drugs most widely used by older people.

With this in mind, we re-examined the distribution of DAR's in Canada reported by Health and Welfare Canada in Table 3.2 to see if the pattern was similar to the distribution of the Canadian population that took more than three medicines within the last two days. The information on medicine taking was obtained from the Canada Health Survey (1981) discussed earlier in this chapter. These distributions are presented in Table 3.3. It can be seen that they are very similar. A Chi-quare test was unable to find a significant difference between them (Chi-square = 3.22, df = 1, p < .1 > .05). This type of analysis can not be taken to mean that taking many medicines concurrently causes DAR's. It does suggest that it is the taking of many medicines at once that puts a person at risk of a DAR rather than age by itself.

Adverse reactions to drugs in the elderly are probably even more widespread than many hospital studies suggest. It seems as though there may well be many such effects that do not come to the attention of a hospital or a physician. In a British study, Martys (1982) interviewed patients in a semi-rural practice about their drug taking, and about possible adverse effects of these drugs. He also took blood samples from each patient to check for digoxin serum levels where appropriate and urea and electrolyte levels. His study revealed that of those taking any drug, 36% were thought to have a possible drug-related symptom or sign that had not previously been detected. This study only examined elderly patients, so comparisons could not be made with other age groups. However, a similar study done by Klein and his associates (Klein *et al.* 1984) on outpatients attending the Johns Hopkins general medical clinics in Baltimore did compare self-reported drug side effects in patients older and younger than 65. Surprisingly, they found

TABLE 3.3

PERCENT DISTRIBUTION OF REPORTED DAR'S IN CANADA FROM 1980 TO 1984 BY AGE AND SEX/EXPECTED FREQUENCY BASED UPON FREQUENCY OF CANADIANS REPORTING USING MORE THAN THREE DRUGS WITHIN THE LAST TWO DAYS

sex	age		total
	less than 65	65+	
male	28.80/23.79	10.96/7.73	39.76/31.52
female	43.54/49.77	16.70/18.70	60.24/68.47
total	72.34/73.56	27.66/26.43	100.0/100.0

Chi-square = 3.22, df = 1, $p < .1 > .05$.

SOURCE: Health and Welfare Canada.

that older patients (25%) reported significantly fewer side effects than younger patients (33%) even though they were taking more medicines. While there are other interpretations of these data, one strong possibility is that older people may be less likely to recognize and attribute adverse effects to their medications than young people. If this were so, it might mean that DAR's may be more likely to be missed in the elderly.

It is also possible that there are many DAR's that are missed even by studies like these because they show up in ways that might not be expected by either the patient, a physician or the researcher. For example, MacDonald and MacDonald (1977) surveyed 390 patients over 65 who had fractured femurs. Nearly all the fractures that had been caused by nocturnal falls occurred to those who were also taking barbiturate sleeping medication at the time. Falls during the daytime were not related to barbiturate use.

Another reason that DAR's might not be detected in the elderly is that many of these effects resemble symptoms that can easily be attributed to "old age" and are not recognized as drug related. Butler (1975) claims that most doctors in practice today believe in what he calls "the myth of senility," that is, that loss of memory, intelligence and the ability to reason is an inevitable part of old age. When it occurs, no other cause need be sought. Drug-produced effects are often missed as a result. Evans and Jarvis (1972) have outlined a characteristic syndrome they have seen in elderly patients taking nitrazepam in doses commonly prescribed by their physician. Some of these adverse effects appeared after the drug had been taken for some time. They noticed that the drug could "unmask" old cerebral damage and lead to an erroneous diagnosis of progressive brain disease. The drug also produced postural hypotension (a fall in blood pressure caused by standing up which sometimes leads to fainting and falling). These symptoms disappeared when the drug was stopped, and there were no permanent effects.

In an Australian study by Learoyd (1972), 236 elderly psychiatric admissions were studied. About 16% had symptoms of disturbed behaviour that disappeared or abated when the psychotropic drugs they had been taking were discontinued. These symptoms included restlessness, paranoia, aggression, confusion, abusiveness and disorientation. Learoyd suggested that this over-medication resulted from attempts by physicians to treat with psychotropic medicines symptoms like moodiness, anxiety, sleeplessness and irritability that result from failing physical and mental abilities. Instead of relieving these age-related symptoms, these drugs often create more undesirable behavioural effects which all too often are treated with still more medicines. This results in patients who are totally incapable of caring for themselves, which in turn creates even more medical problems. Learoyd suggests that this over-medication results in other non-behavioural adverse effects like cerebral and cardiovascular accidents, chest infections and bones broken by falls.

Butler (1985) has suggested that one of the most common reversible causes of dementia in the aged is drug intoxication, and the physicians, when confronted with an elderly patient experiencing a sudden change in cognition, should begin their work-up by stopping all medications. In many cases, he suggests, this will be sufficient to clear the symptoms of senility.

THE NATURE OF DAR'S IN THE ELDERLY

DAR's can be categorized into several types. The most common type seen in all ages is the "augmented" type, that is, the main effect and the side effects are normal, but the drug is administered in an excessive dose that causes an enhancement of the unwanted effect and an unneeded increase in the therapeutic effect. This augmented type of DAR would often be the result of excessive blood levels of a drug caused by the diminished metabolism and excretion that is known to be a result of aging. The agumented type of DAR is preventable with appropriate dosing. Other types are not preventable and include cases where there is an allergy or hypersensitivity to the drug. Such responses are known to occur in a certain proportion of cases, but are frequently not predictable on an individual basis and therefore are difficult to avoid. It has been estimated that 70 to 80% of all DAR's are of the first, preventable type (Melmon 1971). While an extension of this discussion of DAR's can be found in Chapter 6, on prevention and intervention for drug problems, a comprehensive discussion of the nature of DAR's in the elderly is beyond the scope of this book. However, we will discuss the nature of DAR's associated with one representative drug to provide an example of how the elderly are at particular risk. The drug is flurazepam. More complete discussions of other DAR's in the elderly can be found in the following references; Davidson (1985); Melmon (1971); Inciardi *et al.* (1978); and Bressler (1982).

One drug that is commonly prescribed as a night-time sedative hypnotic to the elderly is a benzodiazepine, flurazepam, marketed in Canada under the trade name of Dalmane. As barbiturates are declining in popularity for the purpose of treatment of insomnia, the benzodiazepines are being prescribed more and more. In 1973, flurazepam was the most commonly prescribed hypnotic among hospitalized patients in the United States. In one study, Greenblatt and his associates (Greenblatt *et al.* 1977) report the results of a survey conducted by the Boston Collaborative Drug Surveillance Program which monitors admissions to some hospitals in the United States and Canada. In the years 1970 to 1975, 20% of all people admitted to these hospitals received flurazepam. In nearly all cases, the drug was prescribed for insomnia. Adverse reactions to the drug were noted in 3.1% of all admissions. The adverse reactions were usually unwanted CNS depression causing drowsiness, confusion and ataxia. An analysis of these cases showed that the probability of DAR's increased as the drug dose increased. What is more interesting, however, is that the relationship between dose and DAR was much greater in older patients, *i.e.*, large doses (30 mg or more) were much more likely to adversely affect older people than young people. Figure 3.3 shows this relationship. Doses of greater than 30 mg per day caused DAR's in 39% of those over 70 years, but caused DAR's at a rate of only 2.6% among those under 40. DAR's caused at lower doses were not influenced by the age of the subject to the same extent. Thus, the risk of DAR's in the elderly can be diminished by an appropriate adjustment in dose. It is interesting to note that the *Compendium of Pharmaceuticals and Specialties of Canada* recommends an adult dose of 30 mg, but also recommends that the elderly should be started at 15 mg. The Greenblatt study showed that 28% of patients over 70 had been prescribed the drug at a dose of 15 mg or greater.[4]

CONCLUSIONS

It is apparent that for almost all medicines, both those prescribed by physicians and those that are self-prescribed, there is increased use by older people. While decreased health can explain much of this elevated use, there is strong evidence to suggest that other factors such as perceived health, life satisfaction, stereotyping of the elderly, myths about aging and the like, make a considerable contribution as well.

While there is little doubt that medicines are extremely useful in treating the diseases of the elderly, it is apparent that multiple drug use can also have detrimental effects on health. One of these is that the elderly who take many drugs at one time are much more likely to experience adverse reactions to their drugs. In many cases these adverse reactions cause symptoms such as

FIGURE 3.3

THE FREQUENCY OF ADVERSE REACTIONS TO FLURAZEPAM IN RELATION TO AGE AT THREE LEVELS OF AVERAGE DAILY DOSE

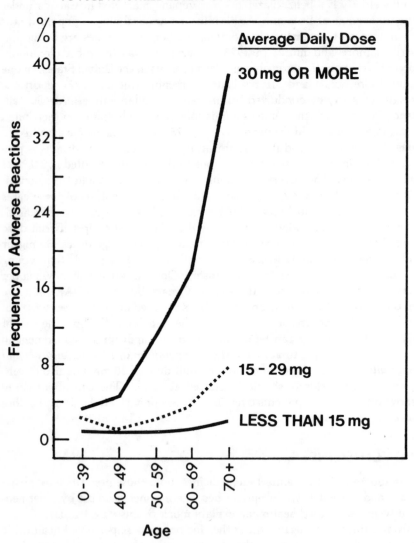

SOURCE: Greenblatt *et al.* 1977. Reprinted by permission.

memory loss, sleepiness, agitation and confusion. All too often these adverse effects are inaccurately diagnosed as being due simply to aging, and may often be treated with even more drugs. There are numerous reports and case histories in the literature that document improvements that result from the stopping of drugs or by reducing dosages.

Quite clearly, the nature and frequency of drug adverse reactions in older people is an area requiring considerably more investigation. As the population of most countries is growing older, these are problems that will become more and more common. It has been pointed out that when new drugs are developed and tested in clinical trials, age is seldom investigated, and old and very old populations are not often used, even though these are the people that are more likely to be given many drugs, and more likely to experience adverse drug effects (Smith *et al.* 1983).

Another result of multiple drug use in older people is decreased compliance to prescribed drug regimens. Most research shows that by far the most common type of non-compliance is under-compliance which, in theory, can diminish the therapeutic effectiveness of drugs. In other cases where the drug is mistakenly taken in too large a dose it can cause adverse drug effects. The actual therapeutic consequences of non-compliance in the elderly, however, have not been intensively investigated.

Before concluding this chapter we should return to the warning by Evan Charney with which we started the section on compliance. It can not always be assumed that lack of compliance, especially drug defaulting, is such a bad thing in the elderly, who seem to be so over-medicated. In a review by Hanlon (1979), it was pointed out that many of the drugs prescribed for the elderly, including maintenance digoxin, are probably unnecessary and can be safely stopped in 70% of cases without any serious consequences (Hall 1973). Hanlon concludes "Until such time as drug therapy is reduced and simplified to supervised administration of long-acting parenteral preparations, at least one swift way to eliminate the problem of non-compliance with some patients is not to prescribe a drug in the first place."

As we have seen, the frequency of adverse reactions to drugs greatly increases as the number of drugs taken increases. It is also not reassuring to read articles like the one by Learoyd (1972) which documents an improvement in psychiatric symptoms in 16% of admissions to a psychogeriatric unit when medication was stopped or decreased. Reluctance to take drugs may be a form of protection against zealous over-prescribing by physicians. Attempts, then, to improve compliance in any population may not necessarily improve the medical status of any patient until they are met by a corresponding improvement in the competence with which physicians prescribe. Considering these factors, we are content to let Charney also have the last word. "... it is probably only an even bet that improving compliance will improve health." (Charney 1975).

NOTES

1. We recognize that the bulk of the literature refers to such effects as Adverse Drug Reactions or ADR's, but we will be using the more modern term of Drug Adverse Reaction here.
2. A Chi-square test is a means of comparing two distributions and determining what the chances are that they are really the same. In this case the chi-square test tells us that the probability that the breakdown of DAR's by age and sex which could be expected in the general population of Canada is less than one in one thousand.
3. We are indebted to E. Napke, M.D., Chief of the Product Related Diseases Division, Bureau of Epidemiology, Health and Welfare Canada, Ottawa, for providing us with this information. These data should not be understood to represent all Drug Adverse Reactions in Canada, but only those reported to Health and Welfare Canada. The information is raw information and has not been scientifically verified by Health and Welfare Canada.
4. In a paper read at a meeting of the Canadian Association on Gerontology, Quebec City, 1986, and in subsequent personal communication, Myrna Baker, Coordinator of Drug Epidemiology for the Upjohn Company of Canada, has reported that in her study of the use of flurazepam by the elderly, 66.9% of prescriptions for flurazepam are for 30 mg. These figures were derived from a postmarketing surveillance study in Canada conducted by the Upjohn Company. The population studied were people over 65 who picked up their own prescriptions from a pharmacist. In this sample, older, chronically ill female patients are underrepresented, so the generality of these figures is not known.

CHAPTER 4

THE RESTORATION AND PRESERVATION OF YOUTH: DRUGS AND ALTERNATIVES

INTRODUCTION

Since the inevitability of aging and death have always been a concern to mortals, it is not surprising that humans have made repeated attempts to slow, stop or even reverse the aging process. In this section we will deal with some of these attempts, but an important distinction must be made at the outset. It is generally believed that there is a theoretical maximum to the duration of life. Most species appear to have a characteristic life span that is predetermined, probably genetically. There have been several guesses at the allotted life span of human beings. The ancient Hebrew Psalmists set this maximum in the Bible (Psalm 90) at three score and ten years, although they conceded that 80 was possible. In the early part of the last century the English mathematician Benjamin Gompertz, who was one of the first to study life-span statistics for large populations, suggested a theoretical maximum of 100 to 110 years. Modern estimates have not changed much. Leonard Hayflick, a modern geneticist, on the basis of studies of the division of body cells, has suggested that the theoretical upper limit is about 110 to 120 years (Kurtzman and Gordon 1976).

In ancient times most members of our species died of disease, war or accident well before they reached the biblical limit, but in recent times, with better medicine, nutrition and sanitation, more of us are avoiding disease and premature death and getting closer to the limits proposed by modern theorists. It follows, then, that aging and the diseases of aging are entirely different phenomena, yet either process can bring the end of life (Comfort 1973; Davidson 1979).

There are basically three approaches to diminishing the effects of age. The first, called the immortalist approach, attempts to extend the maximum upper limit of life and alter the basic process of aging. Immortalist attempts are not aimed at any particular disease. The incrementalist approach includes interventions that extend and improve the quality of life of individuals by treating the diseases and avoiding accidents that are responsible for the deaths of older people, but they do not necessarily extend the programmed age. Finally, there is the meliorist approach that simply tries to

41

improve the quality of life of the elderly by diminishing the symptoms of both old age and the diseases common to the elderly (Parker and Gerjuoy 1979).

Here we intend to deal with all three approaches, although it is sometimes not easy to make these distinctions. The interventions we discuss are not limited to drugs, but also include special diets that both include and exclude substances, and changes in lifestyle. For the most part these interventions, especially the immortalist interventions, arise from some theory of what the aging process is, and as a consequence, we will be discussing these theories along with the treatments.

While the dream of eternal youth has occupied mankind for centuries, the possibility of prolonging the potential for life may not be so difficult to attain. Dr. Alex Comfort, a well-known researcher and gerontologist and director of research on gerontology at the University College of London, speculated that "If the scientific and medical resources of the United States alone were mobilized, aging could be conquered within a decade." (Kurtzman and Gordon 1976). He made that statement in 1973.

CHANGES IN LIFESTYLE

Shunamatism

One ancient view of the nature of aging is that the body is imbued with a certain life force or vital factor like the flame or fire in a lamp. As one ages, this factor is used up and becomes weaker, and when we die, it is extinguished. It was likewise believed that increasing body warmth by eating "hot" foods and by staying warm would preserve vitality. In addition, this vital force could be transferred from the young and vigorous to the old and feeble simply by proximity in the form of body heat. This belief was expressed in the practice of shunamatism exemplified by the aging King David (Kings 1:1) who was brought a young virgin, Abishag the Shunamite, to lie with, when his bedclothes were no longer able to keep him warm at night (Morgan 1981). This technique was also tried by the Roman, Hermippus, who lived to the age of 115 "by the breath of young women" (Davidson 1979).

Many believers in shunamatism felt that sex was not necessary for rejuvenation. As Roger Bacon, a Franciscan friar, mathematician and physician of the thirteenth century, wrote "If disease is contagious, why not vitality?" (Little and Withington 1928). David simply took advantage of Abishag's warmth and did not have sexual intercourse with his young bedmate (Kings 1:4). Among the proponents of the importance of sex, however, was Avicenna, the Arabian physician, who was also fond of this medicine and prescribed it for himself regularly. Laboratory studies suggest that Avicenna may well have been correct. One study with male rats showed that mated rats lived an average of 27% longer than celibate rats (Drori and Folman 1971). Unfortunately, we are not told whether the female rats involved were older or younger than the males, or whether the mating had the same beneficial effect on female rats, although other studies suggest that this may be so (Dunker and Tippit 1973).

With or without sex, it is difficult to say whether there is anything in this theory. Physiologically, there is no vitality factor which can be passed from the young to the old that might prolong life. However, a recent study has shown that men over 50 with wives younger than themselves have a lower mortality rate than those with partners older than themselves (Foster *et al.* 1984). The authors of this research, however, were unable to determine whether this was a result of premarital selection of younger wives by healthier men, or whether the effect was a result of living (and perhaps sleeping) with a younger person.

Exercise

The classical physicians of Greece and Rome believed that one of the best methods for treating the disabilities of old age was by diet and exercise. In addition to warm baths and wine, one of Galen's principles for maintaining health in old age was to maintain activity (de Beauvoir 1972). Modern research supports this ancient theory by showing that exercise has both meliorist and incrementalist, if not immortalist, effects.

Both cross-sectional and longitudinal studies have shown that the capacity for physical work declines with age. For most of the early part of our lives, this decline causes little concern because in our Western civilization the demands placed upon our bodies for physical work are so slight that they are well below our physical capacity. Therefore, this age-related decline is not noticed until we reach the age when even these modest physical demands of daily living approach and surpass our declining capacity. At this point, our lack of physical capacity becomes a severe hindrance, reducing independence and severely diminishing the quality of life. This physical decline in fitness not only diminishes our capacity to meet the demands of daily life, but also decreases our capacity to resist disease.

Is this decline in physical capacity to work and to fight disease an inevitable part of the aging process, or is there anything that can be done to stop it or to slow it down? The answer is quite clear that, to a considerable extent, this decline can be slowed by exercise. Smith and Gilligan (1983) have suggested that half of the decline in biological functioning that reduces our physical capacity is due to lifestyle, specifically, not enough physical exercise. Another researcher (Shephard 1978) has suggested that regular fitness training starting at the time of retirement may delay by as much as eight years the age at which a person is no longer able to cope with environmental demands.

Not only does exercise improve the ability to cope with the demands of life, but it seems as though it has other beneficial effects as well. Fitness programs for the elderly have been shown to improve capacities, including reaction time (Spirduso 1980, and Van Fraechem and Van Fraechem 1977), cognitive performance and memory (Stacey *et al.* 1985). Other studies report improvement in fluid intelligence (Elsayed *et al.* 1980), lower levels of anxiety and depression (Ledwidge 1980) and improved sense of well-being (Stacey *et al.* 1985).

What sort of exercise will be effective in reducing the effects of aging? It seems clear that exercise must be aerobic in nature, that is, it must stress the capacity of the lungs to absorb oxygen and the heart to carry it throughout the body. This sort of effect is usually achieved by continuous strenuous exercise that increases the heart rate to 80% of its maximal rate for at least 20 minutes (Walford 1983), and it must be done regularly.

Most research shows that as people in our society get older, they tend to become less and less active and become less likely to participate in a regular exercise program (McPherson and Kozlik 1980). It seems unfortunate that older people, who stand to benefit the most from exercise, participate less. This may well be a result of cultural expectancies, but the problem of participation may have other sources as well. It has been shown, for example, that a given amount of work will seem to require less and less effort for a young person as he or she becomes increasingly fit, but for older people, in spite of increasing fitness, perceived effort does not decline with practice. If such effects are interpreted by the older person as a lack of progress, it may be increasingly difficult for older people to maintain the motivation to continue in an exercise program. For this reason, it may be necessary to design exercise programs for the elderly that provide a generous measure of social and other rewards for participation. Such a program in St. John's, Newfoundland, the 3-F program (Fun, Fitness and Fellowship), has met with considerable success (Stones *et al.* 1985). For an excellent review of this area see Stones and Kozma (1985).

CHANGES IN DIET

Dietary Restrictions

In 1566, a Venetian nobleman, Lodovico Cornaro, died at the age of 99, and even at the time of his death he was in excellent mental and physical health. In his eighty-third year he wrote a treatise on how to live a long life. One of the major tenets of Cornaro's book was that long life could be achieved by restricting food intake. "The food a man leaves does him more good than what he has eaten." Cornaro's theories were widely disseminated and believed, but he had his detractors. One critic claimed that Cornaro had lived his life as an invalid so that he might die in good health (Vischer 1947).

However, modern research has shown that Cornaro might have been on the right track.

Most reviews of interventions to retard the aging process conclude that the most successful intervention for improving the life span of laboratory animals has been severe restrictions of food. The classic experiment was done in 1935 by C.M. McCay (McCay *et al.* 1935) and has been replicated many times since then in many different species (Rothstein 1982). In McCay's experiment, an experimental group of rats was fed only essential vitamins, minerals and proteins. The control rats were given an unlimited supply of normal rat food. McCay found that the control group lived the normal rat lifespan, with the oldest surviving to 969 days. On the average, the experimental rats lived twice as long as the controls, with the oldest surviving to 1,320 days. McCay's deprived rats were smaller, but they retained vigour and a glossy coat long after the control animals had died. When returned to a normal diet at the age of 1,000 days, they experienced a growth spurt, and many of the females had litters. For a review of McCay's work see McCay *et al.* (1956) and Prehoda (1968). Later experiments have also shown that rats on dietary restrictions not only live longer, but have fewer cancers and other diseases (Tannenbaum 1947; Masoro *et al.* 1980).

The exact relevance of this work for humans has still not been fully developed. Most studies with non-human subjects show that nutritional restrictions have their greatest effect if they are begun very early in life, certainly before maturity (Barrows and Beauchene 1970). It seems unlikely that under-feeding children is going to become popular, but the McCay effect certainly makes a strong case for not over-feeding children. Although most of the benefits of the McCay effect are achieved by restricting the diet during early development, some benefit can still be achieved even if restrictions are not imposed until the later half of life (Stuchlikova *et al.* 1975). McCay himself recommended a diet of Brewer's yeast, whole wheat flour, wheat germ, liver, eggs, milk, calcium and vitamin B1 supplementation. There are a number of published diets that, if followed, could prolong life according to McCay's ideas. Three of these are the Scarsdale diet, the Atkins diet and the Pritikin diet. These diets have been evaluated by Walford (1983), a gerontological researcher at the UCLA School of Medicine, who concluded that the Scarsdale diet, consisting of 1,000 calories a day, with 43% protein, 22.5% fat and 34.5% carbohydrates, comes closest to the regimen described by Cornaro. The diets that increase the life-span of laboratory rats are closer to the Pritikin diet: 10% calories from fat, 10% from protein and 80% from carbohydrates. The Atkins diet recommends high fat, high protein and low carbohydrates, just the opposite of conventional dietary wisdom, and is not recommended by Walford, although he admits that it has not been studied in animals.

Would such diets be likely to prolong life? Possibly. Leaf (1973) observed that the centenarians he studied were lean and tended to eat low-calorie diets. Thomas Parr, who lived to be 152, ate a low-calorie diet of skimmed cheese, milk, coarse hard bread, beer and sour whey. He became famous for his vigour and long life, and a few years before his death he was brought to London and presented to the king. He changed his diet in London and began to eat rich foods and drink fine wines. Physicians at the time believed that his death shortly thereafter was due to this change in diet (Lorand 1911). McGlone and Glick (1978), in their study of persons over 80 in Great Britain, found that of those in the 80 to 90 age group, 114 were classified as thin, 182 normal and 37 as fat. In the 90 to 100 group, 99 were normal or thin and only 10 were fat. They found no persons over 80 whom they could classify as "truly obese." Similarly, actuarial tables indicate that underweight people can expect to live 15 to 20 years longer than those who are overweight (Parker and Gerjuoy 1979), although recently the Metropolitan Life Company of America has increased its ideal body weight tables by 10% (Adelman 1985). It has been concluded that "A moderately slow decline in food consumption to a final level that is two-thirds of the amount normally consumed, supplemented with vitamins and minerals, is certainly feasible in humans, and would undoubtedly produce the largest life-span increase that could be expected from any presently known interventions." (Parker and Gerjuoy 1979).

Dietary Supplements

One widely accepted view of the nature of the natural process of aging is that there is a limit on the number of times a cell can reproduce itself. With increasing numbers of replications, the cell makes more and more errors. As a result, cells formed by later divisions will be less and less vigorous, and after about 50 divisions the newly formed cells can no longer survive. These cells are also more likely to be cancerous. The errors are a result of spontaneous changes in the ability of the genes either to replicate themselves or to control the functioning of the new cell, or changes in the ability of the enzyme systems of a cell to control its own biochemistry. Some theories hold that these errors are programmed in the cell, and that nothing short of genetic interventions are likely to slow the process. However, others believe that the errors are a result of biochemical processes that can be controlled.

There are a number of factors known to cause damage to the genetic and other material in the cell. One is the presence of free radicals, molecules that are created from chemical reactions in the body. Free radical molecules contain an unpaired electron that can combine with and damage other cellular molecules. One researcher has called free radicals the "great white sharks in the biochemical sea" (Walford 1983). Free radicals have many other deleterious effects on cell physiology, including causing damage to the membranes of lysosomes, small bodies in a cell that release powerful enzymes that can also damage much cellular machinery, including DNA.

A number of substances, called "antioxidants" or "free radical scavengers," are known to be able to neutralize or "quench" these free radicals and protect cells from their effects. The body has a number of natural antioxidants, and there are some that can be consumed in the diet. In theory, if these are taken continuously and in sufficient quantities, they should slow aging by reducing free radical damage. These agents include substances that are presently added to food as preservatives such as MEA (2-mercaptoethylamide HCL) and BHT (butalated hydroxytoluene). Vitamins like C and E are natural free radical scavengers that are consumed in the diet either in natural form or as supplements. Another interesting free radical scavenger is ethyl alcohol.

Harman, the developer of antioxidant therapy, maintains that a diet with reduced polyunsaturated fat (a source of free radicals) and increased vitamins C and E may make it possible for a significant number of people to live beyond 100 years. (Kurtzman and Gordon 1976). While it would be nice to believe, there is little evidence to support such a claim. In addition, there is a good possibility that has not been fully investigated that many of these substances like food preservatives have harmful effects at higher doses.

At some time or another, a case has been made for just about every conceivable vitamin as a youth drug. Perhaps the best known are vitamins C, E and B5. Linus Pauling, the only person to have won two Nobel Prizes without having to share either (one for chemistry and one for peace) has been a champion of vitamin C. Pauling reasoned that humans evolved on a diet of fruit that contained enormous quantities of vitamin C. As a result, our bodies lost the ability to make and store the vitamin, and modern man, who consumes comparatively few foods containing vitamin C, experiences a chronic and drastic deficiency which can only be made up by daily ingestion of enormous doses of the vitamin. While vitamin C is Pauling's main vitamin of concern, he recognizes that many other vitamins are also essential. Every day, he personally takes 2 g of vitamin C, 1,200 units of vitamin E, 4,000 units of vitamin A and 50 mg each of several B vitamins.

While vitamins C and E are free radical scavengers, there is no evidence concerning the effects of these vitamins on longevity in humans. Most studies on animals have not shown any increase in maximum life span with vitamin E (Rothstein 1982) or vitamin C (Leibovitz and Siegel 1980), but there is evidence from animal studies that vitamin E might be modestly successful in increasing the number of rats surviving to 24 months. This suggests that vitamin E may be a more effective incrementalist intervention than an immortalist intervention.

Vitamin B5 was discoverd by Dr. Roger Williams while investigating the effect of royal jelly on the life expectancy of bees (Williams 1972). Williams found that B5 increases the life expectancy of mice by 20%. He states that daily doses of the drug from the time of birth might easily be expected to increase life span in humans by 10 years, although there is little real evidence to support this contention.

While the benefits of vitamins as useful interventions for the elderly are debatable, many people take them in enormous quantities, believing that megadoses of water-soluble vitamins can do no harm, but this may not be true for the elderly. Peter P. Lamy (1985) has pointed out that megadoses of vitamin C can suppress leucocyte function, cause the formation of stones in the urinary tract, acidify the urine and aggravate iron overload. One study of the elderly in New York found that nearly 30% were taking vitamins (Chien *et al.* 1978). Similarly, 27% of a population of fit elderly in Edmonton were found to be taking vitamins (Skelton 1985). (See Table 3.1). Other research has shown that 11% of the elderly were taking vitamin C at potentially harmful doses (Lamy 1985).

While agents such as those discussed above are known to neutralize free radicals in the laboratory, it is possible that free radical scavengers may not be doing anything to affect the level of free radical reactions in the cells of a living organism. It has been pointed out that the addition of extra free radical scavengers could have the effect of reducing the activity of the body's natural free radical buffering system, resulting in no change in total activity (Zolier 1985), although there is evidence that the addition of antioxidants to the diet of laboratory animals does slow the accumulation of insoluble pigments that are a result of free radical damage (Leibovitz and Siegel 1980). In addition, neither lifespan-enhancing effects nor meliorist effects have been demonstrated for any of these vitamins or food preservatives in humans.

There are food preservatives that act as antioxidants and serve to protect the components of cells from the harmful effects of free radicals. These substances, such as BHT and MEA are effective as food preservatives for this reason. Animal studies have shown that antioxidants are effective in prolonging life 7% to 29% (Harman 1968), but only when the environment or nutrition was otherwise subnormal (Kohn 1971). These substances are also useful in protecting organisms from the effects of radiation, which are sometimes considered similar to the effects of aging.

Membrane Stabilizing Agents

One of the undesirable effects of free radicals is that they break down the membranes of lysosomes. Lysosomes are tiny packets found in every animals cell that release digestive enzymes which function to destroy unwanted substances in the cell. The membranes of these lysosomes can be damaged by free radicals, and this causes the enzymes to leak out in larger than normal quantities and cause damage to sensitive parts of the cell, including its DNA, and leads to many unwanted symptoms. The drug centrophenoxine is a membrance stabilizing agent that protects the membrane of the lysosomes. Its use in the elderly has resulted in relief from depression and loss of memory, but there is still no evidence that it increases life span (Drestren 1961). Centrophenoxine is not available in Canada.

Yoghurt

Yoghurt has long been regarded as an important dietary contributor to longevity. Even modern television commercials have shown Eastern European peasants, supposedly of great age, who attribute their longevity to eating yoghurt. The association of yoghurt and longevity goes back to the turn of the century to a Nobel Prize winning biologist, Elie Metchnikoff, who speculated that the main causes of old age were alcohol, syphilis and a toxic substance that resulted from bacterial action or putrefaction of food in the intestine. He held that parasitic bacteria in the bowel formed a toxin that was absorbed in small quantities into the body and caused the body to age. In order to slow or prevent this toxin from forming, Metchnikoff proposed a vegetarian diet and the consumption of the Bulgarian sour milk, yoghurt. He claimed that the bacteria that cause the yoghurt to form, *Lactobacillus bulgaricus*, also suppress the bacteria that generate the toxin (Vischer 1947).

In support of his theory, Metchnikoff claimed that Bulgaria, where yoghurt is widely consumed, has a larger than expected population of centenarians, a fact that has more recently been found to be incorrect. Today, Metchnikoff's theory has no scientific credibility; however, yoghurt is still associated in the popular mind with longevity and health, an association not discouraged by the manufacturers of dairy products.

Alcohol

Shunamatism was rooted in the belief that it was the warmth of the young person that served to revitalize the elderly. Warmth could also be acquired by consumption of "hot" food and drink. Ancient physicians believed that wine was such a commodity. In "The Odyssey," Ulysses gives this advice to his father. "Warm baths, good food, soft sleep and generous wine,/These are the rights of age, and should be thine."

The reputation of alcohol as a rejuvenator, or even as a meliorist intervention has declined over the last two hundred years with the rise of the temperance movement and a recognition that alcohol, especially in its distilled form, was responsible for much personal and social harm. More recently, however, the benefits to the elderly of moderate alcohol consumption have been rediscovered. The section on alcohol in Chapter 5 reviews research on the possible benefits of alcoholic beverages for the elderly.

MEDICINES AND THERAPIES

Apart from changes in lifestyle or diet, there have been many other attempts to prolong life and/or cause rejuvenation in the elderly. They can best be thought of as medicinal or therapeutic interventions. The following discussion of some of these is by no means exhaustive. The examples presented here are representative of some of the more extreme and better known attempts and serve to demonstrate the lengths to which people will go, with the help of physicians, to restore youth.

Plant and Animal Materials

Historically, there have been many plants that were believed to possess the power to revitalize the aged. Many of these were primarily known as aphrodisiacs or sexual stimulants, but their regenerative powers were also believed to restore vigour to the aged. It was generally held that sexual potency in males was an index of the life force, and that interventions that increased sexual potency did so in the course of general rejuvenation. In addition, the loss of sexual abilities was a symptom of aging that was of great concern. One such cure was the mandrake root. The mandrake plant has a large tap root that often divides into two branches and takes on a shape roughly resembling the human form. Because of the principle of sympathetic magic, *i.e.*, that like things affect each other, and the fact that the mandrake root contains the anticholinergic, hallucinogenic drugs scopolamine and atropine, the plant was used by witches and sorcerers to make magic potions and cast spells (McKim 1986). It was also used by males as an aphrodisiac. Mandrake roots assisted Jacob to impregnate both of his wives, Lia and the aged Rachael (Genesis 30: 14–16). While it may have nothing to do with the plant's reputation, anticholinergic drugs have been used successfully to treat Parkinson's disease and can improve the activity of the elderly thus afflicted.

Other ancient rejuvenants include soma, the God-drug of the Aryians of Northern India (now believed to be the *Amanita muscaria* mushroom, Wasson 1968), bird's nest soup and ginseng root of China, orchids, and seafoods like oysters and lobsters. Even water itself was thought to have great power to restore youth. Most mythologies contain stories of immersion in water bringing youth, and the search for fountains of youth motivated many explorers, including Ponce de Leon, who discovered Florida in 1513 (Trimmer 1967). A more complete account of the history of rejuvenation therapies can be found in Trimmer (1967) and Segerberg (1974).

Hormones

At the turn of the century it was believed that the symptoms of old age were similar to those of lowered levels of thyroid hormone, hypothyroidism

(Vischer 1947). Subsequent research showed that, indeed, thyroid extracts did improve the condition of many elderly people among whom hypothyroidism was common, but it did not appear to have any effect on life expectancy.

The ancient preoccupation with sexual performance as an index of general vitality showed up in the nineteenth century in a most peculiar form. It has long been believed that the general decline in the well-being of aged males was a result of diminished levels of sex hormones. One of the most remarkable figures in this story is Dr. C. E. Brown-Séquard, a well known professor of experimental medicine. In 1889, at the age of 72, he astonished the medical community when he claimed in a lecture to the Societé de Biologié in Paris that he had succeeded in rejuvenating himself by injecting an extract of dog testicles. He further claimed that the extract permitted him to satisfy his young wife, whom he had recently married. Brown-Séquard's claims were never widely accepted by the medical profession, his young wife soon left him and he died five years later, but he did start a rather long-lived tradition (Trimmer 1967). In the first half of this century there was a flurry of testicle transplants into elderly males in the belief that they would cause rejuvenation. The testicles from both goats and monkeys were used, but neither increased life span, although there was a short-lived period of rejuvenation. Both types of testicles succeeded in making their proponents very wealthy. Unfortunately, the monkey testicles transmitted only syphilis to their unfortunate recipients (Kurtzman and Gordon 1976).

Replacement therapy of estrogen, a female sex hormone, after menopause has been shown to relieve many of the symptoms of menopause, but there is no evidence that it increases the life span. On the negative side of estrogen replacement therapy there appear to be problems with breast cancer and vascular disease in post-menopausal women (Davidson 1979).

Paul Niehan's Cell Therapy

In 1931, Dr. Paul Niehan successfully treated a woman whose parathyroid gland had been accidentally removed. He found that her symptoms were permanently relieved when he injected her with the minced parathyroid gland of a steer. He fully expected that the relief would be short-lasting and disappear when the appropriate hormones from the steer's gland had been used up, but the cure was permanent. Niehan believed that the cells from the steer gland had somehow caused the regeneration of the woman's own parathyroid. He extended this principle to other tissues and the result was cell therapy. Cell therapy is based on the belief that cells from a healthy organ will cause a regeneration of a deteriorating organ when injected. Since old age may seem to result from a deterioration of organs, such injections should cause a general rejuvenation and delay death. This thinking bears considerable resemblance to the rejuvenation principles of shunamatism.

Originally, cell therapy consisted of a urine test which was supposed to determine the functional capacity of each organ in the body. A pregnant sheep would then be slaughtered, and cells from the appropriate organs of the sheep's embryos would be injected into the patient. The technique was later modernized by using freeze-dried organs rather than fresh tissue.

Cell therapy received considerable prominence and was patronized by notables like Somerset Maugham, who lived to be ninety-one, and Pope Pius XII, who lived to be eighty-two. Niehan himself survived until 1971 when he died at the age of eighty-nine. His technique is still being used in Switzerland and in clinics around the world, but it is illegal in the United States and is not practised in Canada (Kurtzman and Gordon 1976). In spite of the notable individuals who ascribed to it, cell therapy has never been scientifically evaluated and has no basis in contemporary science.

Gerovital

Gerovital is procaine hydrochloride, which is also known by the trade name Novocaine. It is a local anesthetic often used in dentistry. It works by blocking the ability of a nerve to conduct information when it is injected nearby. In the 1940s, procaine was being studied by Dr. Ana Aslan, a Romanian physician. Dr. Aslan injected the drug into the arteries of elderly people and found that it relieved the symptoms of vascular disease, angina, asthma and degenerative joint disease. In addition to the relief of these symptoms, she found that there was a great improvement in all aspects of the well-being of her geriatric patients including memory, performance, strength and vitality. Dr. Aslan was so impressed that she called the drug Gerovital and promoted it as an antidote to aging.

In 1951 a new preparation was introduced which was called Gerovital H3 or GH3. The procaine solution was made more stable by the addition of benzoic acid and potassium metabisulphite which also extended its biological half-life. This drug can be given by intramuscular injection. Treatments are given in a series of eight injections, repeated 12 times a year and are administered regularly. It is widely given throughout Romania.

On the basis of clinical trials, Aslan claimed that the drug improves the survival rates of the elderly, but others have disputed this finding (Zwerling *et al.* 1975). Apart from its purported ability to prolong life, Aslan claims that the drug relieves many of the symptoms of old age such as deafness, wrinkles, grey hair and impotence. Once again, these claims are disputed. Gerovital may be useful in the treatment of depression since the drug has properties similar to a class of antidepressant drugs known as monoamine oxidase inhibitors (Cohen and Ditman 1973). Because it is a vasodilator it might also be expected to increase blood flow to various organs, including the brain, and thereby improve their functioning. Such an effect has yet to be demonstrated.

Although many older people flock to European clinics to receive Gerovital injections, there is no convincing independent evidence that this therapy has any immortalist, incrementalist or meliorist properties. For this reason the treatment is not used in clinical practice in Canada, Great Britain or the United States. These countries will not likely permit Gerovital until such time as careful clinical trials reveal any positive effects on physical or mental health.

CONCLUSIONS

After reviewing all of these interventions, it seems clear that the most effective immortalist intervention is selective dietary restriction — not dietary supplements or special additives, but under-eating without under-nutrition. The most effective meliorist and incrementalist intervention is simple physical fitness maintained by regular aerobic exercise. Neither of these interventions depend upon modern medicine or technology, and both involve simple lifestyle changes that have been proposed and successfully practised for hundreds or even thousands of years.

Perhaps the final word of this chapter should be left to Dryden (Cape 1979, p. 276):

Better to hunt in fields for health unbought
Than fee the doctor for a nauseous draught
The wise, for cure on exercise depend
God never made his work for man to mend.

CHAPTER 5

RECREATIONAL DRUGS

INTRODUCTION

Few people pause to think that they are taking a drug when they drink a cola beverage or eat a chocolate bar. Yet, in both cases they are consuming a powerful stimulant, caffeine, probably in significant quantities. Recreational drugs are substances consumed for non-medical reasons. In the previous chapters we considered drugs whose use was motivated by a desire to cure illness, alleviate symptoms, extend life or reverse the processes of aging. This chapter concerns chemicals used non-medicinally for the experience which use of the drugs may produce. Many of the drugs considered in this chapter, such as caffeine and tobacco, form such a part of people's daily routine that users are not frequently aware that they are "using drugs." However, the chemical effects and side effects of these "recreational" drugs often have as powerful an impact upon the user as many prescription medications. With certain drugs, such as in cigarette smoking, the original pleasure or satisfaction which motivated initial drug use may disappear after time although the user remains addicted to the drug. With the elderly, recreational drug-use patterns often began quite early in life, when the original motivations for using the drug were quite different from the experience of the older drug user.

This chapter considers tobacco, caffeine, alcohol and various psychoactive drugs such as marijuana and LSD. We present the facts about the drug effects and their patterns of use among the elderly without moralizing about what older people should or should not use. Nevertheless, the facts concerning certain substances, such as tobacco, are sufficiently clear that the overall message of the section is that smoking is highly dangerous for one's health. On the other hand, the case for alcohol is more complex. Moderate alcohol consumption may be beneficial to one's health and well-being, whereas immoderate drinking is highly hazardous. Although the general hazards of the use of recreational drugs are discussed in this chapter, the prevention and treatment of problems arising from the use of recreational drugs are considered in the following chapter.

CAFFEINE

Caffeine has been consumed by people since as early as Paleolithic times. Although caffeine is present in at least 60 plants, the oldest use of caffeine-containing beverages in historical records is the mention of tea, which was described in a Chinese dictionary in 350 A.D. However, tea is considered to have been mentioned much earlier in written records dating from the Chinese emperor Chen Nung in 2737 B.C., although the reliability of these records is questionable. A caffeine-containing chocolate drink was served to Spanish conquerors by the Aztec emperor Montezuma in 1519, and coffee was introduced into Arabia from Ethiopia between the twelfth and fifteenth centuries.

Caffeine is the world's most popular drug. Most adults and children in the world today use one of the caffeine-containing beverages on a regular basis. Caffeine is a member of a family of drugs known as the *xanthine stimulants* or the *methylanthines*, which occur naturally in a number of plants. Caffeine is consumed in Canada for the most part in coffee, tea, soft drinks, chocolate, and over-the-counter pain killers, cold remedies and stimulants.

A survey (Gilbert 1976) found that 92% of adult Canadians drank coffee or tea or both on the day prior to questioning. Gilbert estimated (1984) that Canadians consume an average of 238 mg of caffeine from all sources per person daily (the equivalent of 2–6 cups of coffee or 4–8 cups of tea, dependent upon the strength of the brew). A cup of instant coffee contains between 29 and 117 mg of caffeine per cup, perked coffee contains 39–168 mg per cup, drip coffee contains 56–176 mg per cup, tea has 30–75 mg, cocoa or chocolate milk has 75–150 total methylxanthines, a one-ounce chocolate bar has 75–300 mg, 12 ounces of Coca-Cola has 45 mg, and 12 ounces of Pepsi-Cola has 30 mg. Over-the-counter analgesics often include added caffeine. For example, an Anacin tablet has 22.7 mg, Dristan contains 16.2 mg, Excedrin 65.0 mg, Pre-Mens 66.0 mg and Vanquish 32.0 mg. Other sources of caffeine include over-the-counter stimulants such as Wake-Up, No-Doz, Ban Drowz (100 mg each) and Vivarin (200 mg). (Gilbert, Marshman, Schweider and Berg 1976; McKim 1986).

There are substantial variations in consumption patterns based upon cultural differences. Gilbert (1984) cites the case of a pregnant woman who was avoiding drinking coffee because of her pregnancy but was unaware of her consumption of 595 mg of caffeine per day from other sources. A study by Farkas (1979) in a community of Canadian native people reported an astounding daily caffeine consumption from tea alone of almost 1000 mg per person. Canada and the United States, with 5% of the world population and no native sources of caffeine, consume 16% of the available caffeine in the world. The average Canadian consumed 4.4 kg of coffee, .9 kg of tea, 1.3 kg of cocoa and 68 litres of caffeine-containing soft drinks in 1982

(Gilbert 1984; Statistics Canada 1983). Canadians drink about the same amounts of coffee as Americans, but consume much more tea (but not nearly as much tea as the British) and less chocolate and cola drinks.

Barone and Roberts (1984) calculated caffeine consumption by age for men and women from coffee, tea and cola drinks. The daily consumption in milligrams was converted to a milligrams per kilogram of body weight measure since the effect of caffeine, like most drugs, is dependent upon its concentration in the body. Women weigh less on the average, so that less caffeine is needed to have the same effect. Furthermore, weight varies with age, and these variations need to be taken into account in order to understand the impact of caffeine consumption on individuals. They found that caffeine consumption from coffee reaches a peak in the 35 to 64 year range, with about 83% of people being coffee drinkers. Although the percentage of coffee drinkers does not change in the 65 to 74 and the 75 and over age ranges, people consume less caffeine (a decline from 3.8 mg/kg age 35 to 64 to 2.9 mg/kg age 75 and over). Although men consume about 15% more caffeine than women, there is little difference in the consumption per kilogram of body weight.

Tea consumption also peaks in the 35 to 64 age range and declines subsequently. However, the caffeine consumption per kilogram of body weight remains fairly constant throughout adulthood (at about 1.1 mg/kg), with no significant sex difference.

Cola drinking differs more markedly with age. Children and adolescents have the highest caffeine consumption per kg (*e.g.*, .88 mg/kg age 3 to 5, .71 age 6 to 8, and caffeine consumption .57 age 9 to 14). Caffeine intake from cola drinks declines to .23 mg/kg for women and .29 mg/kg for men age 75 and over. From age 35 onward the percentage of cola drinkers declines. In the 19 to 34 year-old group 57% of men and 46% of women consume cola beverages. Cola consumption declines to 9% of men and 8% of women in the 75 and over group. This age difference is probably due to generational differences in drinking patterns. Cola drinks have only recently been heavily marketed, with particular emphasis on the youth markets. As the current younger generation grows older it is possible that they will retain their current higher consumption patterns of caffeine from cola drinks.

Caffeine consumption from chocolate and cocoa products is not as well studied as from coffee, tea and cola drinks. Age differences in chocolate consumption are not well documented to date. Accurate data on chocolate consumption patterns would be needed to complete a description of age differences in total caffeine consumption.

After drinking coffee or tea, the caffeine is completely absorbed from the digestive system and reaches peak blood levels between half an hour and one hour later. Caffeine does not generally accumulate in the body for more than a day and has a half life averaging 3.5 hours. Caffeine is mostly eliminated by the liver, and persons with liver damage may retain caffeine in their bodies for longer periods of time.

Caffeine has been shown to improve performance on a number of tasks ranging from athletic activities to visual monitoring (Laties and Weiss 1962). However, the improvements seem to only help eliminate the effects of fatigue. Since many older persons seem to feel more fatigued, many turn to caffeine products to help improve performance. The effects of caffeine are greatest on non-users, with habitual users experiencing less effect. This suggests that a tolerance or habituation phenomenon occurs with caffeine use.

Caffeine consumption has relatively few harmful effects when consumed in moderation. People who consume caffeine may have more trouble falling asleep when compared to non-users and less frequent consumers. Since older persons often experience troubles falling asleep and wake more easily (Mishara and Riedel 1984), caffeine consumption should be evaluated as a possible cause or exacerbating factor when sleep problems are encountered.

Caffeine consumption in the 5 to 10 cups of coffee a day or equivalent dosage range can lead to problems such as flushing, chilliness, insomnia, irritability, irregular heart beat, and loss of appetite (Mosher 1982). Consumption in the 1000 mg range (10 to 15 cups a day) is more likely to produce such symptoms and may produce severe reactions which mimic an anxiety neurosis. When an adverse reaction to caffeine use is to blame for an anxiety reaction, drug therapy is usually not effective; the only cure is to eliminate caffeine from the diet.

Caffeine can interfere with the effects of several psychotherapeutic drugs such as the benzodiazepines *e.g.*, chlordiazepoxide (Librium) and diazepam (Valium), and the antipsychotic drugs in the phenothiazine family, like chlorpromazine.

Further research on the beneficial use of caffeine in the elderly would be warranted to determine under what circumstances and what dosages caffeine may be useful and to ascertain when caffeine consumption is responsible for negative side affects such as restlessness, sleep disturbances and anxiety reactions. Persons working with the elderly should be aware of the possible role of caffeine in these difficulties and should evaluate total caffeine consumption, including the use of chocolate and analgesics which contain significant amounts of caffeine.

TOBACCO

In the early part of the sixteenth century the newly discovered medicinal herb, tobacco (*Nicotiana tabacum*), was greatly proclaimed for its many positive effects on health and well-being. It was not until four centuries later that the extensive negative effects of tobacco use upon health were scientifically proven. In the interim, the smoking of tobacco has become one of the most widespread drug-use activities in human culture. In Canada there are about 6.2 million smokers, with almost a third (32.7%) of all Canadians 15 years of age and over regularly smoking cigarettes (Millar 1983). Canadians have one of the highest *per capita* tobacco consumption rates in the world, and the Canadian tobacco industry has annual sales in excess of 3.4 billion dollars.

The most important chemical constituent of tobacco smoke is nicotine, a fairly toxic substance. As little as 30 mg of nicotine can be fatal, which is surprising, since a cigarette contains 15 to 20 mg of nicotine. However, only a fraction of the nicotine in a cigarette is inhaled by smokers. Nicotine is responsible for most of smoking's negative effects on health. Other important constituents of tobacco smoke are tar, which refers to the particles in the smoke, and carbon monoxide, the gaseous result of incomplete combustion.

The risk of many diseases is increased immensely by smoking (see Van Lancker 1977 for a review of smoking and disease). Smokers are much more likely than non-smokers to suffer from lung cancer, cancer of the mouth and upper respiratory tract, other respiratory diseases such as bronchitis and emphysema, heart diseases, blockage of blood vessels, and stomach ulcers. The heavy use of alcohol combines with smoking to increase the risk of tobacco-related heart diseases and cancer. Women who smoke tend to reach menopause at an earlier age than women who do not smoke.

The various diseases linked to tobacco smoking are quite well documented and result from different components of tobacco smoke. Most of the harmful effects are related to complex interactions between the negative effects of inhaling carbon monoxide and the negative effects of the ingestion of nicotine. Pollin (1977) estimated that in the United States, where there is a smaller percentage of smokers than in Canada, one out of every six people alive today will die prematurely from cigarette smoking. He reported that the elimination of smoking would save 300,000 lives in the United States per year, including a 33% reduction of deaths by heart disease and arteriosclerosis, 50% reduction in deaths from cancer of the bladder, 85% fewer deaths due to bronchitis and emphysema, and 90% reduction in deaths from cancer of the trachea and lungs. Such a reduction would have its greatest impact on the elderly, since most deaths in later life are due to cancer and heart disease. (Young people are more likely to die from accidents and suicide.) (Mishara and Riedel 1984)

Smoking generally begins in adolescence. Adolescents start smoking due to peer pressure, curiosity, desire for status and other social reasons. Thus, most elderly smokers have been smoking for most of their lives (although some had quit temporarily several times in the past). Figure 5.1 shows that there are relatively fewer older smokers, when compared with other age groups. About 15 percent of persons age 65 and older smoke cigarettes

FIGURE 5.1

VARIOUS CATEGORIES OF CIGARETTE CONSUMPTION BY AGE AND SEX IN CANADA

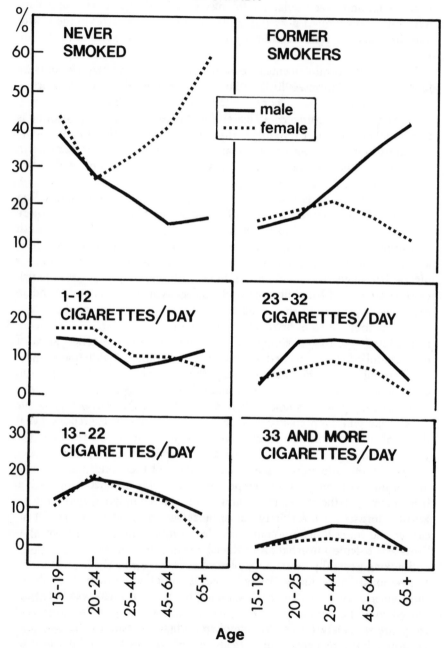

SOURCE: Canada Health Survey 1981, Table 11, p. 50

regularly. This compares with 34% in the age 45 to 64 group, 55% in those age 20 to 44, and 23% in the 15 to 19 year olds. Men are somewhat more likely than women to smoke regularly, with the sharpest sex differences observed in the over 65 groups. This sex difference is probably due to generational differences between people who are now old and young. It was culturally less accepted for women to smoke at the beginning of the twentieth century when the current generation of older persons began their smoking habits as adolescents. Figure 5.2 shows that smoking declined in males between 1966 and 1981, but remained fairly stable for females during this time period.

Why are there fewer older Canadians who smoke? One explanation is that many people stop smoking as they grow older due to concerns about their health. The section on former smokers in Figure 5.1 shows that, at least for the males, a significant proportion (over 40%) had quite smoking earlier in life. Women smoked less frequently than men overall, and those older women who did smoke tended less frequently to quit smoking.

A second explanation for the age difference in smoking patterns is that the negative effects of smoking upon health are so strong that significant number of smokers never survive to grow old. This explanation certainly accounts for some of the age differences, since smoking does have a strong effect upon longevity. For example, the mortality rate of all smokers in the 45 to 55 age range is double the rate for non-smokers in the same age range. Pollin (1977) estimated that eliminating smoking would mean that 33% fewer males age 55 to 59 would die.

Bosse, Garvey and Glynn (1980) examined the hypothesis that smokers tend to develop more psychological and pharmacological addiction as they age. They measured psychological addiction using a scale on which smokers rated their motives for smoking. These motives included smoking for stimulation, smoking for pleasurable stimulation and smoking to reduce negative effect. Pharmacological addiction was determined by measuring the actual amount of tar and nicotine consumed.[1] They found that older smokers did have higher scores on measures of psychological addiction, but did not consume more tar or nicotine than young adults. Longitudinal data over a relatively short three-year time span supported cross-sectional data showing that older smokers tend to "get more out of smoking," in that they express more reasons for smoking on tests of smoking motivation. The authors conclude that although older smokers are more psychologically dependent than younger smokers their pharmacological dependence does not increase, so that they do not consume more tar and nicotine.

A national survey of attitudes towards smoking conducted by Data Laboratories (1978) of 1,006 Canadians in 32 large population centres showed some interesting age differences. Smokers in the age 55 and over group were less likely to want to quit smoking than any of the younger age groups. Persons over age 55 were less concerned about the health hazards than the 25 to 34 year-old groups. Francophones were more likely

FIGURE 5.2

PERCENT OF REGULAR SMOKERS IN THE CANADIAN POPULATION AGED 15 YEARS OR MORE BY AGE AND SEX IN 1966 AND 1981

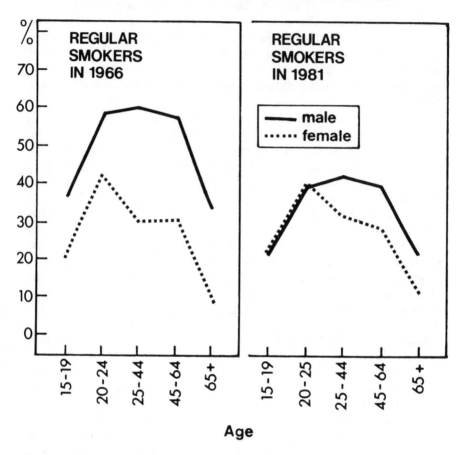

SOURCE: Millar 1981. Reprinted by permission.

than anglophones to smoke, and overall tended to smoke more heavily than anglophones. Although francophones were more inclined to want to quit (72% versus 60%), francophones were more frequently "unconcerned" over the health hazards of smoking (51% versus 22%).

Overall, the findings from this national attitudes survey complement the study by Bosse, Garvey and Glynn (1980). The older smokers in the attitudes survey may be less willing to quit because they have a stronger dependence. However, if we take into account the great percentage of older males who had quit smoking (40%), the results of these two studies may merely be due to the fact that the older Canadians who continue to smoke are those who either are more psychologically addicted or less concerned about their health. A significant proportion of Canadians who smoke seem to recognize the health hazards of smoking as they grow older, and quit.

There is relatively little research on the psycho-social correlates of smoking in the elderly and the motivations of older persons to continue to smoke or to quit. Perhaps studies of the factors related to quitting smoking successfully in older age groups could help generate ideas for aiding younger persons to quit smoking. Surveys of why people quit reveal that the reasons most frequently given are due to disease symptoms. Quitting smoking, even relatively late in life, seems to offer significant health benefits, although certain lung diseases, once acquired, may not be reversible.

ALCOHOL

Beverages containing alcohol have been consumed for several thousand years, with wine being mentioned in some of the earliest written records on Babylonian clay tablets (see Mishara and Kastenbaum 1980 for a complete historical review of alcohol and the elderly). Early historical records referred to the appropriate use of alcoholic beverages by the elderly for either medicinal purposes or to help older persons forget the sorrows of old age. The Bible contains passages recommending the consumption of wine (Proverbs 31:6,7):

> Give strong drink unto him that is ready to perish, and wine unto those that be of heavy hearts.
> Let him drink, and forget his poverty, and remember his misery no more.

The Bible did not specifically recommend wine for the elderly, but since older persons are more likely to perish and suffer certain miseries, wine could be seen as an appropriate consolation to the elderly who approach death or are suffering. Elsewhere in Proverbs, the Bible recognized that the effects of alcoholic beverages are not always positive: drinking too much can lead rulers to (31:5): "forget the law, and pervert the judgment of any of the afflicted." Thus, we find a dual or ambivalent view of the effects of alcoholic beverages. Alcohol was recognized as possessing positive powers when used appropriately, but could pose a dangerous threat when abused. This dual view of the benefits and dangers of alcohol is seen throughout history and is expressed to this day in laws controlling the availability and consumption of alcoholic beverages in Canada. This section considers the effects of alcohol use in the elderly, Canadian drinking patterns, and the extent and dangers of alcohol abuse. The treatment and prevention of alcohol problems in the elderly are discussed in the following chapter.

Contemporary research and historical analysis reveal the dual nature of the effects of alcohol consumption. Benefits are seen for moderate consumption, but severe dangers abound with alcohol abuse. The possible benefits were first reported historically in the medicinal use of alcohol in the treatment of illness, particularly in old age. Although Moslem tradition forbids the consumption of alcoholic beverages for pleasure, alcohol was used by Moslem physicians as a drug throughout the Middle Ages. For example, Avicenna, the tenth-century Persian physician, advised elderly persons to consume as much wine "as they can tolerate," whereas young people should only "take it with moderation" (Gruner 1930). However, not just any wine would do for the elderly. He advised that only old red wine was appropriate for older people; new and sweet wines should be avoided except under certain circumstances.

Wine was often recommended as part of a health regime aimed at extending life and increasing health and vigour in old age (Mishara and Kastenbaum 1980). When Arnaud de Villeneuve invented brandy at the end of the thirteenth century, he was convinced that he had discovered the magic water of immortality which alchemists had been seeking for centuries. He called his discovery, *aqua vitae* ("water of life") and proclaimed that consumption of this liquid would increase longevity, maintain youth and relieve depression. He apparently did not realize at the time that distillation of spirits would lead to a global trend toward the widespread availability of inexpensive distilled beverages with high alcohol contents.

In 1982 Canadians consumed 212 million litres of alcoholic beverages, which corresponds to an average annual consumption of 11.2 litres of pure alcohol per Canadian over age 15, or about 13 drinks per person weekly (Addiction Research Foundation 1984). About half of the consumption was in the form of beer (49%), followed by spirits (37%) and wine (14%).

Figure 5.3 shows the relationship between drinking patterns and age in Canada in 1979. These data indicate that older Canadians consume fewer drinks than younger Canadians, and older Canadians tend more frequently to be abstainers.

How can we account for these age differences in alcohol consumption? First, we need to determine if the lower drinking rates among the elderly reflect a change in drinking patterns as people grow older, or lifelong generational differences in drinking. The data on former drinkers in Figure 5.3 indicate that a significant proportion of older men (10%) and a less substantial percentage of older women (about 4%) were former drinkers who had given up drinking in the course of their lives. Thus, there is evidence that some older persons stopped drinking as they aged, but not in sufficiently significant numbers to account for the large number of abstainers in the over age 65 groups.

A second hypothesis to explain the low prevalence of drinking among the elderly was proposed by Drew (1968; Mishara and Kastenbaum 1980). Drew suggested that the low prevalence of alcoholism in the elderly may be due to the effect of heavy drinking on mortality. Heavy drinking is correlated with the incidence of many potentially lethal diseases such as liver and cardiac dysfunction. Drew reasoned that there may be fewer heavy drinkers in the later years of life simply because most heavy drinkers die younger. It is true that heavy alcohol consumption is related to increased risk of many deadly diseases. Table 5.1 shows the age- and sex-specific death rates from the diagnosis of "Alcohol Dependence Syndrome" in Canada for 1982. These data add some support for the hypothesis that, at least in the males, alcoholism poses an increasing risk to longevity with increasing age. However, moderate drinking has been related to *increased* longevity (*e.g.*, Belloc 1973; Shurtleff 1970). Heavy drinkers may die earlier, but moderate drinkers may live longer. (This greater longevity among moderate drinkers when compared to abstainers is not necessarily related to alcohol consumption, *per se*. Abstainers are a minority group and may have other unique characteristics other than non-consumption of alcohol which could account for the differences in longevity). Although it is likely that some of the decreased prevalence of alcohol consumption among the elderly is due to premature deaths among alcoholics, this explanation can only account for a proportion of the differences observed.

A third hypothesis is that some alcoholics benefit from treatment and quit drinking, accounting for the age differences in alcohol consumption. This hypothesis is probably the least tenable, since outcome results on alcohol treatment programs are inconclusive, and only a small proportion of alcoholics in Canada complete a "cure" of their drinking habits.

Fourth, there is speculation (Mishara and Kastenbaum 1980) that there are generational or "cohort" differences in drinking patterns. That is, older Canadians may have always consumed less alcohol than younger (more recent) generations of Canadians. Perhaps, due to a carry-over from the Prohibition movement in the United States and its parallels in Canada, a greater proportion of members of the older generation have moral beliefs against drinking or just were not raised in an environment where as much drinking was present. There is little evidence for this fourth hypothesis, since sufficient data are lacking to determine the true merits of this explanation.

A fifth explanation is that the data on drinking among the elderly are not as reliable as data from other age groups (Mishara and Kastenbaum 1980). Most data are derived from survey research in which interviewers ask people to tell about their consumption patterns. Old people may tend to more frequently "forget" (intentionally or unintentionally) the exact extent of their drinking or be less willing to reveal that they drink, in order to maintain an image of "propriety." Since current data rely solely upon self-reports, the accuracy of age differences depends upon the accuracy of the original data. It would be useful to obtain more direct measurements of consumption by, for example, examining purchase of alcoholic beverages by different age groups at liquor stores.

As shown in Figure 5.3, women abstain from drinking twice as frequently

FIGURE 5.3

VARIOUS CATEGORIES OF ALCOHOL CONSUMPTION BY AGE AND SEX IN CANADA

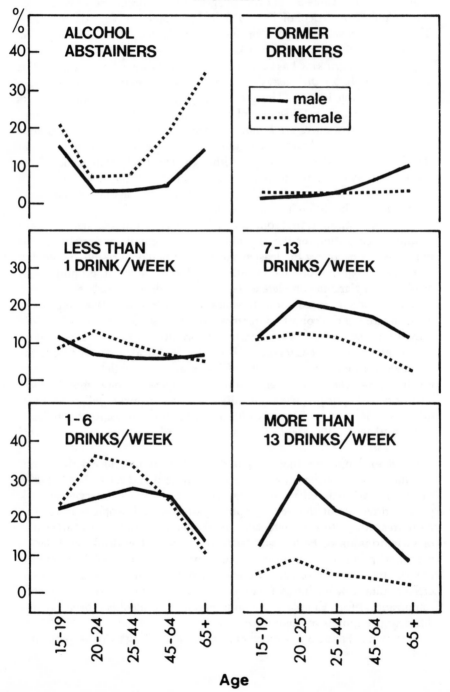

SOURCE: Canada Health Survey 1981, Table 1, p. 28

TABLE 5.1

AGE- AND SEX-SPECIFIC DEATH RATES FROM ALCOHOL DEPENDENCE SYNDROME IN CANADA IN 1982 PER 100,000 POPULATION

age	male	female
under 20	—	—
20–24	.1	—
25–29	.4	—
30–34	.6	.1
35–39	1.4	.3
40–44	3.9	.1
45–49	5.1	1.0
50–54	5.6	4.1
55–59	10.0	2.0
over 60	10.7	1.9

SOURCE: Addiction Research Foundation 1984.

as men, and women drinkers drink less in general. These sex differences parallel differences observed in other countries, but may be changing for the current generation, since the least sex differences occur for the teenage (age 15–19) groups. It is also interesting to note that women aged 20 to 45 more frequently drink less than 1 or 1 to 6 drinks a week, whereas men are more frequently heavy drinkers. Physiological differences in body weight may account for a small part of the reason women drink less: women weigh less on the average and thus require fewer drinks, on the average, to attain the same blood alcohol concentrations as men. However, the data clearly indicate that men drink much more. Unless the data for women are more biased towards under-reporting than data for men, this phenomenon indicates a stable sex difference worthy of further study. One explanation of these differences is the institutionalization of drinking practices for men, with the greater availability of bars and taverns where mostly men congregate to drink. It will be interesting to observe the effects of more recent laws guaranteeing equal rights and opportunities for women upon sex differences in future drinking patterns.

Age differences in alcohol effects have just recently received increased attention in the research literature. As with other drugs (see Chapter 2), responses to ingestion of the type of alcohol present in alcoholic beverages, ethanol (CH_3CH_2OH), varies with age. In general, equivalent amounts of ethanol per kilogram of body weight injected into the blood or ingested orally result in higher blood ethanol levels after absorption (Mishara and Kastenbaum 1980, Chapter 2; Wood 1985). However, the mechanisms underlying the increased blood alcohol levels are not clear. There do not seem to be age differences in ethanol elimination (Vestal, McGuire and

Tobin 1977). It seems most likely that age differences in ethanol blood con-centrations are related to age differences in the proportion of fatty tissue and body water. Ethanol is water miscible but not fat miscible so that ethanol does not distribute to fatty tissues. Figure 2.1 (see Chapter 2) shows that between age 25 and 60 the percentage of total fatty tissues of total body weight almost doubles in men and increases by 50% in women. Since ethanol is limited to distribution in the water compartments of the body, equivalent amounts of ethanol would be more concentrated in older people who have proportionately more fatty tissue in their bodies. Thus, older people generally are less tolerant of ethanol, or, if one desires to look at the positive side, older people need to consume less alcohol to have the same effects as their younger and leaner friends.

Although most of the research on alcoholic beverages has been focussed upon ethanol, it is important to note that there is more to many alcoholic beverages than just their alcohol content. The other constituents, called, "congeners," constitute the hundreds of other substances found in wine, beer, and spirits in quantities varying from microscopic traces to significant proportions of total volume. Beer, for example, contains carbon dioxide, fluoride, hydrogen sulphide, phosphate, sulphur dioxide, calcium, copper, iron, magnesium, potassium, sodium, lactic acids, tannins, amino acids, ammonia, thiamine, riboflavin, panthenic acid, pyridoxine, nicotinic acid, biotin, sugars, maltodextrins, and peptides, just to name a few. The con-geners in wine are even more complex. Because of the congeners in alcoholic beverages, it is possible that research studies, which almost invariably use only pure ethanol, may not provide a complete picture of the effects of alcoholic beverage consumption by people who drink such complicated concoctions as beer and wine.

Like other drugs previously discussed, the effects of ethanol depend upon the rate of administration, the social context, personal variables (such as expectations) and the presence or absence of illness or chronic disease. Tolerance develops with prolonged use, and ethanol also produces cross-tolerance for several classes of other drugs (Eckardt *et al.* 1981). Of par-ticular concern is the dangerous cross-tolerance to sedative and hypnotic drugs such as the benzodiazepines. Combination of ethanol with other drugs is the most frequently reported cause of drug-related medical crises. Adverse reactions include cross-tolerance-related interactions with benzo-diazepines and other minor tranquilizers, *e.g.*, diazepam (Valium), anesthetics, morphine and other opioids, certain antidepressants, anti-hypertensives, anticonvulsants, antibiotics. Furthermore, ethanol can increase the sedative effect of over-the-counter antihistamines and the anti-coagulant effect of aspirin (resulting in massive gastric hemmorhages in alcoholics).

Ethanol is metabolized in the liver and provides about 7 calories per gram. Because of the nutritive properties of ethanol, people who drink heavily may not feel hungry. Malnutrition from lack of proper nutrients is a common problem among alcoholics.

As previously mentioned, moderate alcohol use (less than 2 drinks a day or a total of less than 30 ml of ethanol) does not seem to result in more frequent health problems, according to current research. However, older people may find that the two-drink upper limit needs to be reduced to compensate for the increased blood alcohol levels described above. However, greater consumption is linked to a variety of disorders, with the risk increasing with greater and more frequent alcohol use. Immoderate drinking can result in reduced hepatic (liver) functioning. Cirrhosis of the liver due to chronic drinking is linked to a series of related disorders including gynecomastia, testicular atrophy, spider angiomata and palmar erythema (Gambert, Newton and Duthie 1984). Chronic alcohol ingestion is related to a range of cardiovascular problems including cariomegaly, cardiac fibrosis, microvascular infarcts and swelling and altered subcellular myocardial components (Gambert, Newton and Duthie 1984). Nevertheless, moderate drinking of less than two drinks a day has been related to *reduced* risk of myocardial infarction (Klatsky, Friedman and Siegelaub 1974; Yano, Rhoads and Kagan 1977) and reduced coronary artery disease (Anderson, Barboriak and Rimm 1978; Yano, Rhoads and Kagan 1977). Colditz *et al.* (1985) showed that moderate drinkers are at less risk of death from coronary heart disease, and Marmot *et al.* (1981) showed that there is a slightly lower mortality rate for light drinkers than for either abstainers or heavy drinkers.

The subject of problem drinking will be considered in depth in the following chapter. We conclude this section with a discussion of recent research on the possible beneficial effects of alcoholic beverages upon sleep and well-being in the elderly.

Since 1963, several studies have reported possible beneficial effects from serving wine or beer in moderation to older persons, both in institutions or living independently at home. The earliest studies were conducted by Robert Kastenbaum and his colleagues at Cushing Hospital in Framingham, Massachusetts (Kastenbaum 1972; Kastenbaum and Slater 1972). They found that introducing wine and/or beer in moderation in a geriatric hospital enhanced sociability among geriatric patients and had no adverse side effects. Soon, several other studies were conducted which supported these basic findings and suggested beneficial changes following moderate consumption of alcoholic beverages upon several variables including depression, morale, sleep and participation in activities (Mishara *et al.* 1975). A full range of alcoholic beverages was available instead of just beer and wine, but consumption was limited to two drinks (with equivalent alcohol contents) per day in the experimental group. The beverages were served in a social setting (like in prior studies), but a control group was included who were offered only non-alcoholic beverages in an identical social setting. Other aspects of this study included complete assessments of physical health by physicians before participation and after 9 and 18 weeks (focussed upon changes most sensitive to alcohol consumption such as hepatic functioning and cardiac problems); extended observations over 18 weeks; comparisons of nursing home groups with more independent older persons living in a community residence; and gathering of control data on past consumption patterns and concurrent consumption among the independent community residents.

The results of this study showed no negative effects of the availability or consumption of alcoholic beverages upon the physical health or well-being of the nursing home residents and the more independent community groups. In fact, members of the experimental group who had alcoholic beverages available worried less and the community group had higher morale as assessed on a standard morale scale. In the nursing home, those who consumed alcoholic beverages regularly reported less trouble falling asleep. These effects could be differentiated from an increased socialization which occurred in both experimental and in control groups (which did not have alcoholic beverages available during the first phase of the research). No systematic changes in physical status could be related to alcohol consumption in either setting. The only significant change in health-related variables was a decrease in pulse rate among drinkers, which could be seen as an indication of improved cardiac functioning. This reduction in pulse rate was not associated with any cardiac pathology, and could not be seen as an acute effect of ethanol, since the physical measures were not obtained on the same day when alcohol was consumed.

Overall, the authors concluded that their study confirmed previous research: The moderate use of alcoholic beverages appears to have benefits for those who choose to partake (although not the same benefits for all individuals) and relatively few drawbacks. They warned that these conclusions apply only for situations where proper medical clearance and follow-up are present. Also, the voluntary nature of participation must be assured. In this study, the alcoholic beverages were available, but individuals decided if they wished to imbibe each day. Adverse reactions may have been avoided by a self-selection process whereby older persons who anticipated negative reactions would choose not to drink.

One of the fears of the director of the community residence where this study took place was that, because of the freedom of the participants to leave the residence and purchase alcohol on their own, some people would become alcoholics after participating in the investigation. No evidence of alcoholism induced by the interventions was observed. However, the residents appreciated the social hours so much that, after the end of the study, they petitioned the director to continue those activities on a regular basis.

It is not clear from the Mishara *et al.* (1975) study if the effects observed were directly due to the chemical effects of ethanol or psychological reactions to being treated as a responsible adult by being offered alcoholic beverages in a social setting, or other psycho-social reactions to drinking or participating in a social setting where alcohol is available. Because of the added social benefits of the social setting, independent of having alcohol available, it would be advisable for institutions considering offering alcoholic beverages to their residents to consider doing so in a social setting rather than just including alcohol as part of a formal medication routine.

One of the most persistent findings concerning the institutional use of wine is improved sleep patterns. For example, Mishara and Kastenbaum (1974) found that consumption of wine (containing the equivalent of .4 oz. of ethanol) each evening reduced the need for medications to help their samples of institutionalized elderly mental hospital patients sleep. Mishara and Kastenbaum (1980) speculated that this improved sleep may be related to the presence in wine of gamma-amino-butyric acid (GABA), which is not found in other alcoholic beverages. Kastenbaum (Mishara and Kastenbaum 1980) conducted a series of studies in which he provided wine to older persons living independently in their own homes and asked that they take one or two glasses of wine nightly. Two hundred and thirteen older persons participated in experiments where ten days of pre-wine measures of sleep and cognitive functioning were compared to measures taken after nightly consumption. Most participants (84%) limited their consumption to one glass daily. Self-report measures of sleep quality indicated no negative effects of wine consumption, and there was improvement in significant numbers of participants, most notably after 10 to 15 days of wine consumption. Improvements were noted in mood and morale. Furthermore, there were indications of cognitive improvements in memory tasks after the drinking phase.

Mishara and Kastenbaum speculated that these findings may be due to improved sleep resulting from wine use. They further speculated that the GABA or other congeners in wine may increase the deep Stage 4 sleep, which generally declines in old age. These hypotheses could warrant further investigation by appropriate experimental investigations in sleep laboratories.

Overall, the studies of alcohol and the elderly indicate a double-faced phenomenon. When consumed in moderation (one or two drinks a day maximum), alcoholic beverages do not seem to pose any threat to health or well-being. In fact, a glass or two of wine may improve sleep, increase feelings of well-being and perhaps even help certain aspects of cognitive functioning. However, as with any drug, certain medical conditions and concurrent use of certain other drugs would contraindicate alcohol use by some individuals.

On the other hand, immoderate use of alcohol constitutes one of the surest ways of increasing the probability of illness and a premature death by chemical means, except perhaps for cigarette smoking. Since smoking and alcohol abuse often occur concurrently, the risk of illness and early death among problem drinkers who smoke is quite high. The next chapter discusses the treatment and prevention of problem drinking among the elderly. There is great reason for concern for the consequences of problem drinking. However, drinking moderately does not necessarily lead to problem drinking. The moderate use of alcoholic beverages should not be confounded with the destructive effects of immoderate or problem drinking.

OTHER DRUGS INCLUDING NARCOTICS AND HALLUCINOGENS

This section considers the use of drugs which are illegal to sell and possess in Canada but which are widely used by certain subpopulations of Canadians. Although there has been considerable research on drugs such as LSD, heroin, cocaine and cannabis (marijuana, hashish, etc.) among younger age groups, we are aware of no study specifically focussed upon the use and abuse of these substances among the elderly population in Canada. This is probably because the use of hallucinogens in Canada is a relatively recent phenomenon, affecting for the most part the generations of people who are under age 40 or 50. Narcotics have been more widely available over a longer period of time, and thus in government studies we see some known cases of illicit narcotic use.

A wide variety of hallucinogenic drugs has been available in illegal "street" markets for over 20 years. These drugs, while differing widely in their physiological effects and chemical constituents, all share the characteristic of potentially causing hallucinations or distorted perceptions of reality. Some, such as lysergic acid diethylamide (LSD) are synthetically derived, while others such as psilocybin and psilocin are found naturally, in this case in the mushrooms of the genus *Psilocybe*. Because of the limited data showing significant use patterns among the elderly, readers who wish further information about psychodelic drug use are referred elsewhere (*e.g.*, McKim 1986).

In official statistics from the Department of National Health and Welfare on hallucinogenic drug cases in Canada between 1977 and 1982 (undated report), the oldest age group of persons, aged 50 and over, had the lowest number of new hallucinogenic drug-use cases of any age group. The maximum number of new cases in the age 50 and over group in any of the six years studied was just 4 persons, and the age 40 to 49 group had just slightly more cases (with a peak of 7 cases in 1980). This compares with between 205 and 500 cases per year in the under age 20 and age 20 to 24 groups. These data explain the lack of concern about abuse of these drugs by older persons. However, as the current younger generation ages, it is possible that they will continue their drug-use patterns to some extent. Thus, it is possible that in 25 to 30 years the use of hallucinogens among the elderly may increase significantly. An alternative explanation is that older hallucinogenic drug users do not come to the attention of the government Bureau of Dangerous Drugs. At this time there is no evidence that this is the case.

Marijuana and hashish, which are derived from the hemp plant, *Cannabis sativa*, are not necessarily included among the hallucinogens since their effects on mood and perception are generally not as marked as potent drugs such as LSD. Data on consumption and effects in the elderly are sorely lacking. The negative effects of *Cannabis* use upon health and well-being have not been established. At least, it is clear that *Cannabis* use poses less of a health hazard than the abuse of alcohol. A Gallup poll in 1982 found that 8.8% of Canadians reported using *Cannabis* within the previous 12 months (Addiction Research Foundation 1985). However, most users were under the age of 30.

There is a growing number of reports on the possible therapeutic uses of *Cannabis* and *Cannabis* constituents in the treatment of glaucoma, asthma and nausea caused by drugs used in the treatment of cancer. There are even informal reports that physicians have illegally recommended the use of illegal marijuana to cancer patients suffering from severe nausea as a side effect of chemotherapy. It is hoped that research will soon reveal the scientific usefulness of *Cannabis* for such purposes and appropriate modifications of government laws pertaining to the availability of this drug will be made, if warranted.

Narcotics include the opiates derived from the Asian poppy, *Papaver somniferum*, and various synthetic related drugs. According to Canadian law, other non-opiate-related drugs such as cocaine (which is derived from the leaves of the *Erythoxylon coca* bush) are included under their classifications of drugs as "narcotics." The opiates with confirmed medical uses, such as morphine, are discussed elsewhere, in the chapter on prescription drug use. Here, we consider the non-medically prescribed uses of "narcotics" such as the self-administration of heroin or cocaine procured illegally.

In 1982 there were 15,295 illicit users of narcotic drugs in Canada, according to government reports (Addiction Research Foundation 1985). These statistics are based largely upon reports from pharmacies, treatment centres and police reports. Thus, they constitute an underestimate of actual narcotic use, since they include only people who seek or get treatment for a narcotic abuse problem and people who get caught by the police. People who do not receive treatment or are not caught by police are not included in such reports. Age differences in the treatment of narcotics abusers will be discussed in the next chapter. Here we limit our discussion to a presentation of some of the effects of narcotics, as well as data on their use in Canada.

Like most drugs, the effects of narcotics depend upon the dosage, previous use patterns, drug dependence, and the circumstances under which the drugs are taken. Regular opiate use results in dependency, and tolerance for these drugs tends to develop. The effects of a single dose appear almost immediately after administration. At higher doses opiates produce a dreamy state where the user is described as being on the "nod" and during which there are vivid dreams and a sense of well-being or euphoria. However, experienced users often report that they take the drug only in sufficient doses to postpone withdrawal symptoms. At higher doses, the respiratory centre of the brain stem is depressed and breathing becomes slow and shallow. Death can result from suffocation in cases of extreme overdose.

Cocaine, which is usually ingested by sniffing in powder form, is a central nervous system stimulant. It produces a brief feeling of euphoria accompanied by a sense of increased energy, alertness and sensory awareness. In too large a dose bizarre sensations can occur, and continued long-term use can result in restlessness, insomnia, excitability and paranoid thinking. Dependence often occurs with regular and frequent use, but tolerance effects have not been conclusively established in humans.

Table 5.2 shows official rates of narcotic drug use in Canada by age groups in 1982. This Table combines heroin, cocaine and other drugs which the government classifies as "narcotics." One may speculate that among the older age groups there may be a higher proportion of heroin and illegal morphine use than among the younger age groups, where one might expect proportionately more cocaine use. This is due to the relatively recent availability of cocaine and the limitations of cocaine availability due to its high price in illegal markets. Older persons may have been introduced to heroin or morphine earlier in life, whereas cocaine use is less likely to have been part of their cultural experiences when they were younger. Furthermore, because of demographic differences between the young and the old in the distribution of wealth in Canada, younger people may be more likely to possess the excess cash needed to sustain a drug habit involving cocaine.

CONCLUSIONS

According to available data, older persons are less likely to use recreational drugs than the present generation of younger age groups. This is probably due to a combination of factors, including the wisdom which leads people to reduce or stop their consumption of certain recreational drugs as they grow older. For some, the motivation to drink less or stop smoking may come more from fear than from wisdom: a heart attack or other medical emergency leads to the medical recommendation to eliminate or reduce drug habits which pose a risk to one's health. In other instances, the older generation never had the experience of using certain drugs as much as more recent generations. For example, marijuana and psychedelic drugs such as LSD were never a significant part of social practices when the current older generation were young. Perhaps the older generation is more reluctant to try these chemicals which receive such adverse publicity in the

TABLE 5.2

AGE AND SEX DISTRIBUTIONS OF THE ILLICIT NARCOTIC DRUG USER POPULATION IN CANADA IN 1982

Characteristic	number	% of total
Sex:		
male	11,996	78.4
female	3,299	21.6
Age:		
under 20	204	1.3
20–24	2,277	14.9
25–29	5,303	34.4
30–39	5,576	36.5
40–49	1,029	6.7
50–59	339	2.1
60 and over	127	0.8
unknown	440	2.9
Total	15,295	

SOURCE: Addiction Research Foundation 1984.

popular media. One could also speculate that the age differences in use of these drugs reflect marketing differences or age differences in abiding by the law.

Since older persons commit fewer crimes, they would thus be less likely to use controlled substances whose sale and possession are illegal. Also, there have been no known attempts to market these illegal drugs to the elderly. One could even speculate that such a marketing decision would not be wise, since the elderly have a relatively low income, obtain free psychotropic medications from physicians, and would therefore be unlikely candidates for spending a few hundred dollars on a small quantity of illegal cocaine, for example.

The recreational drugs older persons use are for the most part legal, easily obtainable and inexpensive. Cigarettes, alcohol and caffeine constitute most recreational drug use. All three drugs may affect older persons more than younger persons, so that less of the drugs may be required by the elderly to have equivalent effects. The mechanisms involved in these age differences have not been adequately researched. Concurrent medical problems, which are more likely to be present in the elderly, complicate attempts to distinguish between age changes and the effects due to specific diseases or changes in bodily components, such as the percentage of fatty and lean tissues. Individual differences are greater in old age. One older person may get "high" on two glasses of wine, while another will feel no effect whatsoever.

What we know about recreational drug use in the elderly is based upon survey studies, whose reliability may be questioned. Older people may not admit to interviewers the full nature and extent of their use of recreational drugs. It would be useful to try to validate present findings on recreational drug use in Canada by seeking corroborative data based upon direct observations of consumption patterns, or patterns of sales in the case of alcohol and tobacco. As we point out in the following chapter, in the case of alcohol there is evidence that under-reporting in survey studies may be quite common.

Physicians, as well as other health and mental health workers, need to pay closer attention to drug interactions with caffeine and alcohol. In the case of alcohol, the results of adverse drug interactions can be lethal. With caffeine, it is important to consider the daily consumption of caffeine (including chocolate and cola beverages) when sleep disorders or anxiety and "nervousness" are present.

Alcohol constitutes a special case, since one cannot generalize about the effects of alcoholic beverages. When consumed in moderation, no negative effects can be noted, and several studies point to benefits for sleep and well-being. However, when alcohol is abused, the effects are often disastrous. The link between moderate use at one stage in life and alcohol abuse at another stage needs to be further studied. Some problem drinkers stop drinking as they age; other moderate drinkers develop alcoholism problems in the later part of life. Both these life patterns need to be further understood in order to help older people who have problems and better understand the mechanisms leading to different drinking patterns in the population in general.

Although we have some data on caffeine consumption rates, we know relatively little about the processes involved in personal patterns of use of this drug. Caffeine offers individuals the potential for changing their psychological state in a rapid, inexpensive and often effective manner. When do older people decide to have an "extra" coffee or two to be more alert and awake and under what circumstances do older people reduce their habitual coffee intake to "tone themselves down"? Psychologists could speculate that depression and expectations about the demands of the moment may influence caffeine consumption behaviour. However, it could be hypothesized just as well that caffeine consumption is related more to long-standing habits than situational or psycho-physical demands. Clarification of the nature of this process could help in the understanding of other processes involved in how older people react to internal physical and psychological as well as external socio-environmental changes.

Despite the long lists of the negative effects of abuse of drugs discussed in this chapter, the overall impression is fairly positive. At the present time, abuse of recreational drugs constitutes a less frequent problem than with other age groups. Nevertheless, the findings presented concern the present generation of older people when studied in the early part of the 1980s. Gerontologists recognize that generational differences can be quite powerful, even in such "basic" areas as intelligence (Mishara and Riedel 1984). Also, older people can adapt quickly to changing mores under certain circumstances. The recreational drug-use patterns in future generations and future times may differ from those reported here for elders living in the first part of the 1980s.

NOTES

1. We speak of consumption of tar and nicotine rather than numbers of cigarettes smoked since cigarettes vary greatly in the amounts of tar and nicotine they contain, and consumption varies as well due to smoking patterns (*e.g.*, length of puffs, depth of inhalation, number of puffs and smoking down to the butt or not, etc.).

CHAPTER 6

PREVENTION AND INTERVENTION FOR DRUG PROBLEMS

INTRODUCTION

This chapter considers what can be done to prevent the occurrence of problems related to the use of drugs and how to help individuals with drug-related problems. The chapter follows the classic typology of dividing efforts to prevent and alleviate drug problems into primary, secondary and tertiary prevention. After a brief presentation and comparison of these three levels of prevention, the specific categories of drugs previously discussed in this book will be considered in terms of possible prevention and intervention strategies. We also include a discussion of two topics which warrant special attention: native people in Canada, and the alleviation of pain in the terminally ill.

PRIMARY, SECONDARY AND TERTIARY PREVENTION

Primary prevention is aimed at inhibiting the development of problems before they begin. Primary prevention problems may focus upon the entire population or certain target groups which are identified as having a higher risk of developing drug-related problems. Primary prevention programs may take different forms, including: advertising concerning the risks of certain hazards (*e.g.*, cigarette smoking), increased monitoring of prescription medications, better labelling of over-the-counter drugs and programs aimed at eliminating causes of unhappiness which may lead to drug abuse. In all these programs, the primary goal is to reduce the incidence of new cases of drug-abuse problems.

Some primary prevention programs are aimed at controlling or improving the system of dispensing and prescribing drugs, such as physician awareness programs and better pharmaceutical packaging. Other primary prevention programs place the emphasis on the drug consumers in helping them have more appropriate drug-taking behaviours or helping them recognize signs of problems.

Although primary prevention seems like a logical starting point for eliminating drug problems in the elderly, relatively few resources are spent in primary prevention activities. This is partly because we live in a society which tends to *react* to problems which seem important rather than anticipate future problems which are preventable. Another reason for the relative lack of emphasis on primary prevention is the difficulty in evaluating outcomes. In primary prevention, the problems one is trying to eliminate are not yet present. If the program is successful, the problems will not occur or will occur less frequently. If the program is unsuccessful, the problem will continue to occur or increase in frequency. It is assumed that between the time the intervention occurred and the results are evaluated, intervening events (*e.g.*, changes in societal attitudes and practices) do not influence the drug-related behaviours in such a way as to confound the effects of the prevention activities. However, this assumption is almost impossible to verify. We live in a changing world in which it is difficult to disentangle prevention efforts from other social changes. Still, primary prevention remains the most cost effective method of reducing drug problems, and, as we shall see in the discussions of specific programs, primary prevention programs are often relatively inexpensive and easy to conduct.

Secondary prevention is aimed at reducing the prevalence of drug problems; that is, the goal of secondary prevention activities is to eliminate or reduce the frequency of occurrence of drug problems which currently exist. As with primary prevention, secondary prevention can be focussed upon the problem itself or the causes of the problem in a person's life (or both). For example, "curing" an alcoholic may involve physical detoxification and treatment in a specialized centre. However, it may be just as important to eliminate the social roots of the problem — the life circumstances which "drive the person to drink."

Tertiary prevention refers to efforts to reduce the impact of a drug problem upon the life of the person and upon society. In tertiary prevention there is no attempt to stop the problem behaviour. The goal is to manage the behaviour or make it less destructive for the person and for society. An example of tertiary prevention is the legal prescription of narcotic drugs by physicians in England. Obtaining legal prescriptions for narcotics allows an addict to obtain controlled dosages of less risky drugs and thus avoid supporting a criminal black market whose high prices provoke criminal behaviour on the part of the addict, who must obtain large sums of money to support the habit. Another example of tertiary prevention involves the appropriate use of addictive pain medications with the terminally ill. Here, the goal is to render life more comfortable for the patients rather than to cure the patients of their problems.

In the sections which follow, we will consider primary, secondary and tertiary prevention as they apply to various types of drug problems. As we shall see, the identification of target populations for prevention activities poses a challenge to persons interested in conducting prevention programs at each level. Furthermore, because of a relative lack of research on the effectiveness of interventions with this age group, the choice of methods of prevention is more often based upon common sense and speculation than firm scientific data.

PRESCRIPTION DRUGS

The prevention of problems involving prescription drugs can occur at several levels of primary and secondary prevention. In primary prevention, possible problems are avoided by appropriate drug-use practices. In secondary prevention, health care professionals and patients may learn to recognize problems when they occur and take appropriate corrective actions. Various groups may be involved in the prevention of problems concerning prescription drugs, including: physicians at the time of prescription and in subsequent diagnosis and monitoring; pharmacists and pharmaceutical companies in the marketing, packaging and dispensing of medicines; the government in policies related to the availability and use of drugs as well as information concerning medications; and the individual and members of his or her entourage at the stages of procuring medications as well as compliance with prescribed routines and identifying possible side effects.

Since prescription drugs are prescribed by a physician, a discussion of possible prevention strategies might well begin with a consideration of how drug problems may be avoided by changes in physician behaviours in both their prescribing practices with the elderly and their communications to elderly patients when drugs are prescribed. Lamy (1985) identified several possible types of drug misuse in the elderly: (1) active misuse or abuse due to over-prescribing, unjustified or inappropriate prescription; (2) passive misuse or abuse, due to lack of re-evaluation of need; (3) the non-use of alternative treatment methodologies (heat, fluids, etc.).

'As shown in Chapter 2, because of age differences in the elimination and distribution of different drugs, special cautions need to be taken when prescribing for the elderly. Unfortunately, specialists in geriatric medicine are rare, and physicians often lack extensive training in geriatric medicine as part of their medical school training. Lamy (1985) warned of the importance of taking into consideration the decreased clearance of several commonly prescribed drugs. These include:[1] Acetaminophen, Aminopyrine, Amobarbital, Antipyrine, Digoxin, Dihydrostreptomycin, Indomethacin, Kanamycin, Meperidine, Phenylbutazone, Phenytoin, Sulfamethizole and Warfarin. He warns that physicians need be aware of the pharmacokinetics of the drugs under consideration, which may be altered in the elderly. A further problem concerns adverse drug interactions. Several authors have attempted to facilitate the identification of potential adverse drug interactions by providing lists or guides which are relatively simple to use. For example, Simonson and Sturgeon (1979) provided an "alert" list of 20 drugs most likely to result in adverse drug interactions. A physician prescribing any of these medications is recommended to evaluate carefully the risk of adverse interactions before prescribing medication from that list. Since adverse interactions may be more likely among the elderly, perhaps physicians should take extra care to evaluate drug interaction potentials with elderly patients. Goldberg (Whiting and Goldberg 1977) developed a cardboard disk where drugs in current use could be compared to alert the physician to potentially dangerous combinations. We are not aware of the existence of similar aids specifically adapted to prescribing for the elderly. The development of such simple tools may help reduce the frequency of adverse drug interactions in the elderly.

Because of the potential for adverse drug interactions, several physicians have questioned the use of polypharmacy (the prescribing of several different medications for the same person). Older people generally take several different medicines each week, with estimates of 14% taking an astounding figure of between seven and fifteen different medications weekly (Lamy 1981). Mishara and Wexler (1986) found that elderly Montreal residents living independently as heads of households took an average of five different medications on a weekly basis, often including several medications for the same disorder. At the present time, there is no control in Canada of multiple prescriptions by different physicians. A central, computerized, record-keeping system to monitor dispensing of medications could help alert physicians to concurrent drug use by a patient.

Certain drugs may pose special problems due to their narrow therapeutic index. Lamy (1985) felt that six categories of drugs widely used with the elderly posed a particularly great threat of misuse due to the small differences between a therapeutic dose and a dose which is likely to produce adverse reactions. These drugs include: (1) anticoagulants, (2) anticonvulsants, (3) antidepressants, (4) antihypertensives, (5) digitalis glycosides, and (6) hypoglycemic agents (oral).

In Chapter 3, we reviewed the problem of compliance with medication routines. The studies we reviewed showed that the nature of the doctor-patient communication affects compliance. Lampe (1985) blames much of non-compliance upon mis-communication between the physician and patient. He cites research showing that it is not "a good bedside (or deskside) manner" that counts, but the quality of the specific information provided concerning the drugs which have been prescribed.

One way to guarantee that important information is provided to patients concerning drugs is to give patients specific Patient Medication Instruction sheets (PMIs), such as those provided by the American Medical Association for certain drugs. The Canadian Pharmaceutical Association, in co-operation with the Health Protection Branch of Health and Welfare Canada, provides Supplementary Information on Medication sheets (SIMs) to medical practitioners and consumers. These sheets describe in a simple, comprehensible manner the purpose of the medication and warn the patient to inform the doctor if other drugs which may react adversely with the medication are taken, or if other symptoms or conditions are present which may indicate hazards or side effects. Further information is given about missing a dose, precautions to be taken and side effects which should be reported to the physician. Similar Patient Advisory Leaflets (PALs), developed by Dorothy Smith, are provided by Pharmex Ltd., Scarborough, Ontario.

A "Medical Information Leaflet for Seniors," printed in clearly readable large type, is provided by the Pharmacy Service of the American Association of Retired Persons. Although the effectiveness with the elderly of such information leaflets has not yet been clearly established, it seems likely that providing such information may constitute an effective means of primary prevention of problems with prescription drug use. It is generally left to the discretion of individual physicians or pharmacists to provide patients with information leaflets. Given the relative low cost of providing such information leaflets, it may be useful to consider a government-sponsored program of drug information specifically focussed upon the elderly, in which information leaflets are provided systematically to all prescription drug users.

When patients leave hospital, they are suddenly faced with the responsibility of organizing what is often a complex regime of pill-taking. In order to help patients cope with medication routines, the Edmonton General Hospital has instituted a self-medication program as part of the patient's discharge planning. In this program, selected patients are given responsibility for administering their own medications with guidance and supervision in preparation for the time when they will have to take care of their medications themselves at home. Such a program is of obvious benefit to people of all ages, but could be especially beneficial to elderly people who are taking many drugs concurrently.

The use of psychoactive medications by the elderly has received particular attention. Parry, Balter and Cisin (1971) suggest that much of our current data on the use of psychotropic medication by the elderly may be invalid due to a pervasive tendency towards under-reporting or lack of reporting in survey studies on drug use. In their studies, 27% of subjects had invalid or only partially valid reponses to drug-use survey questionnaires with regard to the use of sedatives. Rates of invalid responses were higher for stimulant users (33%) and lower for users of tranquilizers (17%). Regardless of the validity of the survey findings on psychoactive drug use, this class of drugs is recognized by several researchers as one of the major causes of adverse side effects.

Often, the side effects are attributed to over-medication. Baker (1985) provides the general rule of thumb that psychotropic drugs should be prescribed as doses only 30 to 50% as large as those for younger adults (see also

Thompson 1983a, 1983b; Salzman 1982). Table 6.1 presents some common side effects associated with psychotropic drug use in the elderly (based upon Moran and Thompson 1982 and Stotsky 1970).

It is assumed that appropriate prescribing practices as well as providing appropriate information when drugs are prescribed can serve to prevent most adverse reactions from psychotropic drug use. Nevertheless, studies show that a very small minority (2 to 4%) of patients ask questions about their prescription while in the physician's office and only six percent receive written information from their doctors (Olins 1985). Furthermore, persons over age 60 are half as likely as younger patients to be counselled about directions for using medications, and younger patients were three times as likely as older patients to ask questions about their medications. Ley (1979) studied patient recall of communications with the physician regarding medications. He concluded that communication practices are often not adequate to insure dissemination and retention of important information. He suggests that, rather than asking questions which can be answered by "yes" or "no," (*e.g.,* Are you taking your medication regularly?) physicians should ask open-ended questions, such as, "When did you last take your medication?" Because patients are often reluctant to ask questions, it is important to create an environment where questioning is openly encouraged.

In addition to improving communication practices, written memory aids should be given, such as dosing calendars, and drugs should be packaged in calendar packs. The effectiveness of giving elderly patients either a tear-off calendar or a tablet-identification card as a memory aid was evaluated by Wandless and Davie (1977). The tear-off calendar contained a personalized list of daily medications and the times each should be taken. The tablet-identification cards had the medications fixed to a card on which the medications were identified, and the times they should be taken were indicated. A third control group received the same instructions as the other groups but did not receive any special medication aids. The tear-off calendar group made fewer medication errors than those with cards, and both experimental groups made significantly fewer errors than those given only standard instructions. Because of the general problem of compliance by elderly patients, these and other aids to medicine use should be considered as adjuncts to standard medical and pharmaceutical practices.

The issue of compliance is complicated by the fact that several people are involved in medication use: the doctor, pharmacist, patient, and members of the patient's family and entourage. Hammel and Williams (1964) found that about three percent of written prescriptions are not even filled within ten days. Current studies of compliance rely on self-reports, which have questionable reliability. Studies involving pill counting seem more reliable, since one can calculate if the appropriate number of pills are missing from the container at any given date. However, missing pills do not necessarily mean that the pills were taken by the patient at the appropriate time. For

TABLE 6.1

POSSIBLE ADVERSE SIDE EFFECTS OF
PSYCHOTROPIC DRUGS IN THE ELDERLY

Class of Drug	Possible adverse side effects
Most psychotropic drugs	Increased daytime sedation
	Expect severe adverse reactions at night. Increased confusion, irritability
Antianxiety agents	
Benzodiazepines	Depression, delirium, confusion
Barbiturates	Habituation, delirium
Sedative hypnotics	
Benzodiazepines	see above
Chloral hydrate	Agitation, insomnia, excitement
Barbiturates	see above
Antihistamines	Delirium
Antidepressive agents	
Tricyclic	Anticholinergic, includes cardiovascular toxicity, delirium pseudodementia, orthostatic hypotension
Monoamine oxidase inhibitors	Hypertensive crises in combination with tyramine and other sympathomimetic drugs
Antipsychotic agents	
Phenothiazines, halperidol	Extrapiramidal movement disorders, restlessness, parkinsonian like reactions, tardive dyskinesia, orthostatic hypotension
lithium carbonate	Delirium, coma, thyroid dysfunction, renal dysfunction, gastrointestinal tremors

SOURCE: Moran and Thompson 1982; Stotsky 1970.

example, a study comparing tablet counts with physiological measures of consumption of antacids among ulcer patients (Roth, Caron and Hsi 1975) showed a 36 percent discrepancy between the two indications of compliance. Studies of compliance in the elderly must go beyond self-reports and pill counts to understand *why* people fail to comply. Although explanations are not lacking (*e.g.*, poor memory, fear or experienced side effects, poor communication of instructions, etc.), further research is needed to test the validity of alternative explanations for compliance problems in the elderly population.

The prevention methods discussed in this section involve both primary and secondary prevention. Primary prevention involves all the activities on the part of physicians, pharmacists and patients to insure that the patient receives the proper medications and appropriate information to permit proper use of the prescription drugs. Secondary prevention occurs when drug problems, such as side effects, are recognized by physicians or patients and proper remedial actions are taken. Other primary and secondary prevention activities are possible outside of the doctor-pharmacist-patient interaction. For example, the Faculty of Pharmacy of the University of Manitoba offers a drug information service, the Medical Information Line for the Elderly, to provide information and counselling for elderly persons and concerned family and friends about medication, adverse drug reactions, side effects, drug misuse and drug interactions.

The Sandy Hill Health Centre in Ottawa has developed a "Medication User's Health Diary" to aid both patients and physicians in keeping track of medications and other important information that could alter the effects of drugs. This diary is a small booklet about the size of a passport in which all medicines, both prescribed and over-the-counter, are recorded along with the prescribed schedule for taking the drugs. There is also space for recording additional information including other substances, like alcohol or caffeine, that should be avoided. In addition, the diary also keeps track of allergies and immunizations and other information that could aid a physician in avoiding drug interactions and in diagnosing an adverse drug reaction.

In our discussion of the prevention of problems related to prescription drugs, we started our analysis with a discussion of physician prescription practices and how improvements may be made. However, we did not explore the basis of physicians' practices. Some critics point to the lack of sufficient training in geriatrics in medical schools. Another possible culprit is the advertising drug companies use to convince doctors to prescribe their products. Smith (1976) conducted an analysis of how the elderly are portrayed in prescription drug advertising. He found that advertising in two major medical journals "tended to reinforce negative stereotypes of the elderly." The written descriptions of the elderly were generally negative, with the more negative descriptions portraying the elderly as aimless, apathetic, debilitated, disruptive, insecure, hypochondriac, having an insatiable need for reassurance, low self-esteem, out of control, sluggish, reclusive and temperamental. The more positive descriptions (which were clearly in the minority) viewed older persons as, her old self, grandmother, respectful and trusting. Although the implications of such content analyses of advertising are open to speculation, one cannot help wondering what influence these descriptions may have in reinforcing negative stereotypes of the elderly, which can lead to less than desirable prescription practices.

One important and neglected aspect of the training of people who work with the elderly is the identification of adverse drug effects. As demonstrated in Chapter 3, adverse effects of many medicines resemble symptoms normally ascribed to "old people," and are often easy to overlook. Such symptoms as memory loss, confusion, sleepiness, even agitation and aggression, are commonly reported for many of the drugs used by older people. Considering traditional stereotypes of the elderly, it is not surprising that such symptoms might go unrecognized in an older person, but be immediately noticed in a 20-year-old. It is therefore important for those who work with older people, especially physicians, to be trained to recognize when drugs are having adverse effects.

DRUGS TO CONTROL PAIN IN CANCER PATIENTS

A current controversy of particular concern for the elderly surrounds the effective management of pain in persons suffering from cancer. Since older persons have a high probability of eventually suffering from cancer, and are likely to die from either cancer or heart diseases (Mishara and Riedel 1984), they may be particularly concerned by the current debate over the availability and use of narcotics such as heroin and morphine in the treatment of cancer pain.

In 1984, a government advisory committee on the management of severe chronic pain in cancer patients completed a report to the Minister of National Health and Welfare (Advisory Committee on the Management of Severe Chronic Pain in Cancer Patients 1984). In that report, they explained that the management of pain in cancer patients who suffer from severe chronic pain may not be adequate due to a number of factors, including the need for improvement of practices involving opiates and other drugs as well as psycho-social supportive measures. They cite:

— erroneous belief that dependence (addiction) need be a clinically important problem with the use of opiate analgesics in cancer patients with pain,

— administration of inadequate dosages of opiate analgesics usually due to inappropriate fear of addiction or respiratory depression, or ignorance about effective analgesic doses,

— administration of excessive dosage, so that patients are free of pain but sedated to the point that they cannot effectively interact with their families or friends,

— use of inappropriate dosage schedules and method of administration including "as required" dose scheduling,

— unnecessary and repeated use of intramuscular or subcutaneous injections of analgesics when a higher dose of oral medication would be adequate,

— failure to administer analgesics often enough and at regular intervals (by the clock) to maintain the patient in a pain-free state,

— failure to increase or decrease analgesic dosage in response to individual need,

— inadequate utilization of non-opiate classes of drugs,

— failure to assess adequately and deal with the complex non-physical factors contributing to the patient's "total" pain experience, and

— failure to utilize appropriate other available adjuncts to pain control which may be useful in selected cases, including radiation and endocrine therapy, nerve blocks, chemotherapy, the use of epidural and intrathecal drugs, palliative surgical procedures, transcutaneous electrical nerve stimulation, acupuncture and a variety of relaxation techniques.

The committee did not feel that the availability of heroin would be warranted at this time, since research has shown that appropriate dosages of morphine are equally effective. They identified certain "entrenched" attitudes and behaviours in the health care professions which need to be changed in order to develop effective control of chronic severe pain. These include the fear of creating "addicts" among the terminally ill, which is unfounded and arises from insufficient knowledge about the actual risks and mechanisms of addiction. Often, the severity of the patient's pain is underestimated and misunderstood due to lack of utilization of accepted methods for objectively quantifying pain. Furthermore, the psycho-social aspects of emotions and suffering may be viewed as unimportant or are ignored. Likewise, ethnic, religious and social attitudes towards pain may be misunderstood or not taken into account.

The committee recommended improved and increased education and training in effective pain management at the levels of the undergraduate professional education of physicians, in post-graduate medical training, and in continuing education of medical, nursing and para-medical personnel. In addition, they recommended that information in the form of a pamphlet be disseminated to the general public about modern pain control measures in cancer. Special pain treatment services need to be developed as well. Finally, more scientific research is needed to develop new drugs for pain control, to test the effectiveness of existing medications, and to help understand individual variations in responses to treatment for severe chronic pain.

Since the Advisory Committee submitted its report, the federal government has approved the use of heroin for certain types of cancer pain (Health Protection Branch 1985). Heroin may only be prescribed for persons who are inpatients or outpatients of a hospital, and the drug remains in the possession of the practitioner or an agent of the practitioner who is administering it to the patient.

OVER-THE-COUNTER MEDICATIONS

As described in Chapter 3, most older persons use over-the-counter medications, and 80 percent of elderly over-the-counter medication users also use prescribed medications, alcohol, or both (Guttman 1978). The elderly use four times as much over-the-counter medication as younger people. Problems associated with OTC drug use in the elderly include adverse interactions with alcohol or other medications, dependence, toxicity and side effects. The primary prevention of OTC drug problems involves efforts at avoiding inappropriate consumption of OTC drugs. Secondary prevention efforts include the recognition of problems arising from OTC drug use and the taking of appropriate actions (usually reduction or elimination of use of the OTC drug).

As with prescription medications, physical changes associated with aging affect the risk of adverse reactions to OTC drugs. Moreover, OTC drugs often contain ingredients which are added to make consumers feel that the drug is having an effect, such as alcohol and caffeine. Regular use of OTC drugs containing these ingredients can produce physical dependence, since once people stop using them, the symptoms for which they were taken come back even stronger than before. OTC drugs prone to such a "rebound effect" include sleeping aids, laxatives and nasal decongestants.

Probably the most effective means of preventing problems associated with OTC drugs would be to better inform the users about the benefits and risks of taking specific OTC medications for the perceived problems at hand. Primary prevention activities could be focussed upon the older users themselves. People tend to take OTC drugs on the basis of self-diagnosis. Drugs are purchased on the basis of expected helpfulness, which may be based upon advertising promises, advice from physicians, pharmacists and friends, past experiences with the drugs and individual decisions to purchase products based upon the appearance of the packaging in a pharmacy or information contained on the package. How can consumers be made more aware of the possible dangers of OTC drug use? The answer to this question is complicated by our lack of scientific data on the relative importance of the various influences on the choice of using OTC drugs. Chien *et al.* (1978) found that most OTC medications were self-prescribed, with significant numbers of OTC drugs reportedly having been suggested by physicians. They found that vitamins, analgesics, cough and cold medications and antacids were among the most "irrationally" used OTC drugs.

Older persons frequently use analgesics such as aspirin and acetaminophen, often because of arthritis symptoms. In a study by Caranasos *et al.* (1974), aspirin led all drugs as a cause of hospitalization. Overdoses can produce acute metabolic disturbances and symptoms of organic mental disorders. The most common dangerous side effect is gastrointestinal bleeding. Aspirin can interact dangerously with several drugs. Cupit (1982) stressed that the major dangers lie in interactions with oral anticoagulants, methotrexate, probenicid, and sulfinpyrazone. He advises that physicians avoid prescribing or recommending aspirin to patients using these drugs, as well as ethyl alcohol, ammonium chloride, antacids, oral diabetic agents, corticosteroids and heparin sodium.

Although aspirin and acetaminophen are both safe for most patients when taken in recommended dosages, acetaminophen is sometimes preferred for some patients, such as those prone to bleed. Cupit (1982) advises that interactions between acetaminophen and chloramphenicol indicate that the combination of these two drugs should be avoided, or carefully monitored.

Gerbino and Gans (1982) warned of the dangers of excessive use of antacids and laxatives for symptomatic relief in the elderly. They stress the need for effective communication to help the elderly make proper product selections, use these drugs appropriately, and avoid complications and adverse interactions with other drugs. Not all antacids have the same acid neutralizing capacity, and several have quite high sodium contents. The high sodium content would be an important factor to consider for persons on a salt restricted diet. Lamy (1982) listed the amounts of the "silent" ingredient, sugar, in various antacids. Twenty products had over 100 mg of sugar per unit, and four had 2,000 mg of sugar or over per unit (per 15 ml or per tablet). This high sugar content must be taken into consideration whenever antacids are prescribed or recommended. Antacids may affect the absorption and elimination of other drugs. Gerbino and Gans (1982) list the effects of oral antacids on the absorption and elimination of 17 different commonly used drugs in the elderly. Because of these effects, elderly persons who must have consistent absorption of drugs such as digoxin, tetracycline, iron salts, levodopa (L-dopa), or isoniazid, should probably avoid simultaneous administration of antacids. They recommend regimens which provide a two-hour interval between the use of antacids and other agents.

Laxatives are used by about 30% of persons over age 60 on a regular basis. Gerbino and Gans (1982) state that people who have taken laxatives for many years have two "mistaken beliefs." The first is that laxatives are safe, and the second is that their actions are confined solely to the bowel (p. 584). They stress the importance of distinguishing between the different types of constipation found in the elderly, and the different types of laxative preparations. Kofoed (1984) warns that the phenolphthalein laxatives are the most likely to cause problems. Laxatives are quite varied, and can be categorized as stimulant laxatives, saline or osmotic cathartics, emollient laxatives, bulk-forming laxatives, enemas and suppositories. Abusers often go to great lengths to hide their laxative habits, rendering diagnosis of laxative-related disorders extremely difficult. Abuse problems are often reflected in hypoalkemia and other metabolic disturbances.

Laxatives are chosen, recommended and prescribed for the treatment of constipation. Most often, the effective treatment of constipation need not involve drugs. Appropriate changes in diet and exercise often eliminates symptoms. Furthermore, there is evidence that, at least in some cases, psychological factors may be responsible for constipation. Greiner, Bross and Gold (1974) conducted a double blind study on patients suffering from chronic constipation. They found that placebos produced improvement in 14 out of 20 subjects. Thus, an effective treatment of constipation (in some cases) may constitute alleviation of the stresses in a person's life or improvement of the coping mechanisms the individual uses to handle stressful situations.

Other commonly used OTC medications include decongestants, antihistamines and anticholinergics. Nasal decongestants produce rebound effects (Kofoed 1984) which may lead to years of abuse. Adverse reactions to sympathomimetic drugs (such as ephedrine and phenylpropanolamine) found in many OTC decongestants suggest that some decongestants should be used with caution by older persons with vascular diseases and persons taking antihypertensive or monoamine oxidase inhibitor drugs.

Antihistamines and anticholinergics, which are common in cold, allergy and OTC sleep medications, can dangerously augment the sedative effects of alcohol, antidepressant medications, antipsychotic drugs and prescription sedatives and hypnotics. Thus, extreme care should be taken when these drugs are taken in combination.

Given the significant potential for problems associated with OTC drugs, how can effective prevention programs be developed? Any efforts at increasing the awareness of physicians, pharmacists and consumers of OTC medications of the nature of OTC drugs and their possible benefits and risks would be a step in the right direction. Such primary prevention activities might include advertising by government or non-profit agencies in which the complications, interactions, side effects and proper indications and contraindications of use of OTC medications are clearly explained. Each year the pharmaceutical industry spends millions of dollars trying to convince consumers to buy their products. Because of their objective of selling their wares, the medications are usually presented as glorious remedies to a wide variety of woes which people invariably experience. Perhaps these biased advertising campaigns need to be counterbalanced by an intensive advertising campaign aimed at providng non-biased information which warns of possible dangers and helps consumers and health professionals to recognize the danger signs associated with OTC drug problems so that they can avoid misuse.

ALCOHOL

Alcohol problems constitute a major social issue which concerns all age groups in our society. As we have seen in Chapter 5, older persons tend to drink less than younger age groups and suffer less frequently from alcohol-related problems. Despite major methodological problems involved in obtaining reliable data on drinking patterns (see Mishara and Kastenbaum 1980), a major problem concerns the criteria used to diagnose a drinking problem. Carruth (1973) examined the constellation of eight symptoms which could be used to identify persons with drinking problems:

1. Symptoms developed as a result of drinking, such as debilitating hangovers, blackouts, memory loss and the "shakes,"
2. Psychological dependence on alcohol, defined as the inability to conduct normal everyday tasks without drinking or planning one's life around drink,
3. Health problems related to alcohol use,
4. Financial problems related to alcohol use,
5. Problems with spouse or relatives as a result of alcohol use,
6. Problems with friends and neighbours as a result of alcohol use,
7. Problems on the job as a result of drinking,
8. Belligerence and problems with police or the law as a result of drinking.

Although these criteria appear to be quite useful with younger drinkers, problems arise when an attempt is made to use these same symptoms with older persons. The "typical" physical symptoms which develop as a result of drinking are quite similar to symptoms which are often associated with "natural" aging. When older persons' hands shake, or they suffer memory losses and are occasionally confused, one does not immediately look for an explanation outside of the normal processes of aging. Health problems are much more common in later life and are often considered a part of the normal aging processes. Thus, health problems are unlikely to be viewed as indications of a possible drinking problem.

Older persons who are retired would not have job-related drinking problems, nor would psychological dependence come to the attention of friends and relatives if the older drinker leads a somewhat isolated existence. Research shows that older drinkers tend to drink at home rather than in public taverns and bars. Because of their more solitary drinking patterns, they would be less likely to have problems with the police, friends, neighbours and relatives. Since older persons tend more frequently to be widowed, problems with spouses are less frequent, and older persons may tend to become more introverted or depressed when they drink when compared to younger drinkers.

Because of the many problems associated with the diagnosis of drinking problems among the elderly, it is often difficult to identify target populations for various prevention programs.

Mishara (1985) presented a model of the development of alcohol problems in old age which differentiates between persons who had lifelong drinking problems (so called, "chronic" problem drinkers) and persons who began to have drinking problems in the later part of their lives ("acute" problem drinkers). Figure 6.1 depicts possible models of the development of alcohol problems in later life. Various individual characteristics determine early life identification of individuals as abstainers, occasional drinkers or acute alcoholics. People who are now members of the older age groups in

FIGURE 6.1
MODELS OF PREVENTION AND TREATMENT OF ALCOHOLISM IN THE ELDERLY

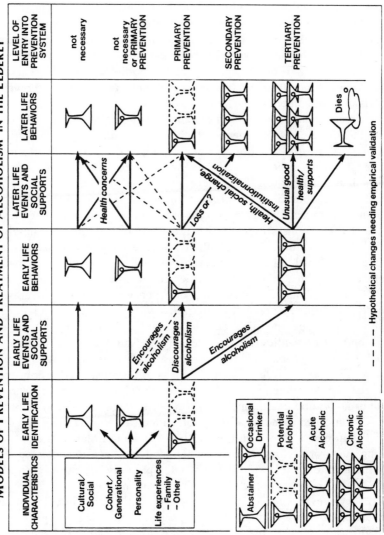

SOURCE: Mishara 1985. Reprinted by permission.

our society had quite different childhood and adolescent experiences related to drug and alcohol consumption when compared to members of the current generations of younger people. As noted earlier, these differences, which are related to the generation or time in history when people were born, are referred to in the gerontology literature as, "cohort" differences.

Research shows that people who identify themselves as abstainers early in life tend to maintain lifelong patterns of abstention from alcoholic beverages. Occasionally, based upon a physician's recommendation, abstainers may drink a bit in their later years. However, there is no indication that significant numbers of abstainers turn to the bottle later in life. Therefore, abstainers are not usually considered a target population for prevention efforts to avoid alcoholism.

Moderate drinkers, on the other hand, depending upon a variety of factors, including early life events which foster or inhibit problem-drinking patterns, may either continue to be occasional drinkers without alcohol-related problems or become acute alcoholics earlier in life. Many early alcoholics never make it to old age since alcoholism poses a significant risk to health (see Chapter 5). Some problem drinkers cut back on their consumption or give up drinking as they grow older due to concern for their health, social changes or institutionalization (people in institutions may simply not be allowed to drink). Acute alcoholics who become occasional drinkers, and potential alcoholics who never developed alcohol problems because they never experienced life events which could foster an alcoholic problem, constitute the principle target groups for primary prevention programs. The objective of primary prevention programs with the elderly is to reduce the number of persons who might develop alcohol problems in their later years.

Secondary prevention is aimed at helping "cure" acute alcoholics who develop alcohol problems in their later years. Most often, the alcohol problem develops as the result of a loss — loss of a spouse, loss of job, etc.

Tertiary prevention activities focus upon the chronic alcoholics who, due to unusually good health and social supports, manage to survive into old age. Chronic alcoholics are a hardy lot, capable of withstanding decades of society's attempts to reform them. Although some isolated cases of long-lasting cures of lifelong chronic alcoholics have been documented, most chronic alcoholics tolerate treatment attempts only insofar as they allow them to return to the bottle after the cure is completed.

Primary prevention activities can focus upon the entire population, as in the case of nationwide advertising campaigns, or specific target populations of high-risk groups. Primary prevention can begin before old age, as with preretirement planning, or in early old age. Some feel that the best primary prevention activities would involve a general betterment of the lot of older persons in Canadian society. An alternative approach would be to focus upon certain crucial life events, such as retirement and death of a spouse, when special supports are needed to cope effectively with difficult circumstances.

Primary prevention activities have the advantage of nipping the problem in the bud, before an alcohol problem becomes rooted in the person's life. Programs can include education about coping with certain life problems, information about drinking and its effects, consultation to help anticipate and avoid problem situations and social changes to better the lot of older persons in society. If primary prevention programs are successful, the incidence of new cases of alcohol problems will be reduced. Unsuccessful programs would not result in a reduced incidence of problems, or else they could result in an increase in alternative problems, such as dependence upon psychotropic medications.

Secondary prevention activities focus upon new problem drinkers, with the goal of bringing about a cure, that is, a permanent elimination of the drinking problems. Secondary prevention activities are hampered by a common mutual conspiracy to deny the nature and extent of the problem on the part of the older problem drinker and his or her family and friends. This pattern of denial often results in a "tardy referral syndrome" whereby help is not sought until it is absolutely necessary, often due to a medical crisis exacerbated by or caused by alcohol consumption. This syndrome, as well as the problems of identification and diagnosis of alcohol problems mentioned above, probably account for the fact that relatively few older alcoholics in Canada receive treatment. For example, Table 6.2 shows that during 1982–1983, the age 65 and over groups had the lowest rate of treatment services for alcoholism of any age group (Addiction Research Foundation 1984). Older alcoholics were invariably treated in hospital-based inpatient facilities. Younger persons were over twenty times as likely to be treated in non-residential programs than persons age 65 and over.

Why are relatively few older persons receiving treatment for alcohol problems, and why is treatment mostly limited to inpatient facilities? Several answers to this question are possible. First, it may be that older persons are less likely to need help for alcohol problems. However, because of the problems in diagnosis, the tardy referral syndrome and tendencies to look elsewhere for the roots of alcohol-related symptoms, it is possible that many older alcoholics are not receiving the help they need. Several authors (see Mishara and Kastenbaum 1980) feel that the lack of treatment, particularly in non-residential settings, is symptomatic of a general lack of non-residential psychiatric and psychological services for older persons, regardless of the nature of their problems. This may be due, in part, to a widespread prejudice on the part of mental health practitioners that older people are harder to help and don't benefit as well as younger clients from psychological intervention.

To date, research on the effectiveness of interventions with the elderly

TABLE 6.2
TREATMENT AND CASELOAD FOR ALCOHOL AND DRUG ABUSE BY AGE IN ONTARIO, 1982–83

Age	Hospital-Based			Community-Based			Total Number
	Detox	Residential	Non-Residential	Residential	Non-Residential	Assessment/Referral	ARF* Community Centre	
	(%)	(%)	(%)	(%)	(%)	(%)	(%)	
Under 18	2.2	3.1	27.3	6.1	20.0	12.1	2.9	3,533
18–29	16.2	32.9	25.3	31.7	42.6	30.9	35.3	13,721
30–49	60.8	45.2	35.5	47.0	28.0	40.8	48.8	28,987
50–64	15.0	16.6	11.5	12.7	8.5	13.8	12.4	7,866
65 and over	5.8	2.1	0.3	2.5	1.0	2.4	0.6	2,265
Total No.	31,361	7,691	2,125	6,073	7,039	1,913	170	56,372

* ARF = Addiction Research Foundation

SOURCE: Addiction Research Foundation 1984.

has shown that older persons benefit at least as well as younger persons from a wide range of psychotherapeutic interventions (Mishara and Riedel 1984). In terms of the treatment of alcoholism, older alcoholics seem to fare better in treatment than younger patients. For example, Linn (1978) found that older alcoholics were more likely than younger patients to remain in treatment. Helzer, Carey and Miller (1984), in a five- to eight-year follow-up of treated alcoholics, found that there was evidence of good outcome in a larger proportion of the older subjects. In another study (Blaney, Radford and MacKenzie 1975) elderly patients had a higher improvement rate in six-month follow-up than younger age groups.

It may be that greater improvement in older age groups reflects differences in the selection of older persons for treatment. Since older persons receive help less often, perhaps those who are finally able to participate in treatment are more highly motivated than younger persons. Nevertheless, there is no evidence to date that older persons do not benefit from help as much as younger age groups.

Tertiary prevention involves helping chronic problem drinkers who have either had a lifelong history of alcoholism, or who have become "chronicized" in later life. Chronic alcoholics hardly ever seek help because they decide to quit drinking. They invariably come into contact with treatment agencies when they have a medical crisis, their living situation or other social supports fail, or the police or other social agencies insist they they get help. Chronic alcoholics have often resisted years of attempts by experts to rid them of their drinking problem. To do so takes a keen sense of survival tactics in order to outwit the health and social services system and stay alive as a member of a marginal subgroup of society. The major problem in treatment is often the inherent conflict between the client's goal of surviving to drink again, and the institutional goal of curing the alcoholic forever. Although most organizations claim to try and cure chronic alcoholics, this goal is probably not very realistic. More appropriate goals would be to prolong the interval between "cures" or institutional stays, to improve the physical health of the alcoholic and the quality of his or her life, and to avoid permanent institutionalization.

ALCOHOL PROBLEMS AMONG NATIVE PEOPLES

Thus far, we have considered drug problems in the elderly population in general, without considering cultural or ethnic differences in patterns of use and abuse. Although ethnic and cultural differences in alcohol use are widely documented, little is known about cultural variations in older Canadians. With respect to the use and abuse of prescription and OTC drugs, we have not found a single research study which studied cultural differences in Canada. The only Canadian subpopulations which have been studied to any great extent are native peoples. The interest in native peoples has focussed upon the problem of alcoholism. This interest stems from the fact that native people have an extremely high incidence of alcohol-related problems.

Although reliable official statistics are not generally available, it has been estimated that between 50 and 60 percent of Indian illnesses and deaths are alcohol related (Indian and Northern Affairs Canada 1980). Most of the concern for alcohol-related problems has focussed upon younger age groups who seem particularly prone to violent deaths and premature illnesses related to alcohol abuse. Up to age 65, native people have a rate of violent death which is three times the national average. Native people have extremely high rates of incarceration in prisons due to alcohol-related offences (Schmeiser, Heumann and Manning 1974). For example, in the Northwest Territories alcohol abuse has been considered to have reached epidemic proportions. In 1974, the number of times people were held over-night in jail by the R.C.M.P. in the N.W.T. because of intoxication was equal in number to one-third of the entire adult population (Canadian Foundation on Alcohol and Drug Dependencies 1977).

In the past, several authors speculated that the alcohol problems among native people might be due to differences in alcohol metabolism. Recent research (*e.g.*, Bennion and Li 1976) has found no differences in alcohol metabolism attributable to differences between Indian and white people.

Several studies of drinking patterns among native people suggest that age differences may exist in drinking practices. Curley (1967) reported that younger Apache drinkers tend to drink in groups of five or six, while older men drink in twos and threes. Curley (1967) and Lemert (1954) suggested that high-ranking individuals, such as chiefs, shamans and public officials, were expected to refrain from drinking. Clairmont (1963) reported that, in an Eskimo community in the Northwest Territories, older people tended to drink in homogeneous ethnic groups, but younger persons would drink in ethnically mixed groups.

There are not sufficient data on drinking among older native people to allow for more than speculation on the implication of possible age differences in drinking patterns among native people. It is clear that mortality rates among native people due to alcohol-related accidents and illness are so incredibly high that significant numbers of native people never survive to old age because of alcohol-related problems.

Explanations of drinking among native people have focussed upon biological models, anxiety models, cultural practices and spiritual explanations. As previously mentioned, current research evidence does not support biological explanations of drinking problems. The anxiety models have received mixed support. Some authors feel that drinking allows native people to release anxieties and aggression brought about by the stresses in everyday life, including the stresses due to loss of native culture and the pressures to adopt national cultural practices (*e.g.*, Dozier 1966). Other authors (*e.g.*, Lemert 1954, 1958) stress the social function of drinking to help develop a sense of group solidarity in the face of white society and a sense of continuity with traditional culture.

One of the problems in discussing prevention strategies among native peoples concerns the value issues involved when judgments are made concerning the behaviours of other cultural groups. Several reports suggest that the major causes of alcohol abuse problems are to be found in the frustrations felt by native people who attempt to achieve economic and social goals which are valued by the dominant society and the difficulties in maintaining a meaningful cultural identity in the face of pressures to change. Further research is needed to better understand drinking among native people and the role of older members of native societies in drinking patterns. Such research might profit from beginning with the point of view of the native people involved. Furthermore, support could be given for native people to develop appropriate prevention programs which attack the roots of the problems, as they see them.

OLDER NARCOTICS ADDICTS

Available data indicate that illegal drug use among the elderly is limited almost entirely to marijuana and heroin. There are no reliable Canadian data on marijuana use among the elderly, although there are a few case reports of use of this drug, and a limited number of older persons admit in survey studies to having "tried" marijuana. However, a number of older heroin users can be identified in Canada. Statistics on drug use (Addiction Research Foundation 1984) recorded 127 known elderly narcotics drug users in 1982, which constitutes less than 1 percent of all users. Studies in the United States show similar figures for narcotics use. However, Winick (1962) observed that people tended to "disappear" from government files between the ages of 35 and 45. He concluded that there exists a "maturing out process" resulting in a cessation of addiction as a result of either the addict's age or the number of years the addict has been addicted.

The idea of maturing out has not been supported in several longitudinal studies which followed addicts for relatively long periods of time. For example, O'Donnell followed up 266 former patients of the Lexington Hospital treatment programs. Of the 21 persons remaining addicted to drugs in the follow-up, only one was recorded as an addict in government records. Capel and Peppers (1978), in a study of addicts who participated in methadone maintenance programs in the New Orleans area, found that ten years after treatment over half of those over age 60 still alive and outside of prisons were still on the active rolls and undergoing treatment. They observed that the number of older addicts is increasing (it more than doubled from 1969 to 1976), and with each coming decade we should expect increasing numbers of older heroin addicts.

Musto and Ramos (1982) challenged the notion that heroin addicts invariably die young or give up their habits. They followed people who were enrolled in a New Haven, Connecticut morphine maintenance clinic from 1918 to 1920. They found that these addicts did not generally die from their addiction, but lived to comparable ages as persons from similar social class backgrounds. DesJarlais, Joseph and Courtwright (1985) explored the survival of older addicts in detail by interviewing older patients in New York City methadone maintenance programs. They interviewed 286 patients between ages 55 and 59, 282 patients between 60 and 69, 53 patients between 70 and 79 and five patients between 80 and 86. Most people were addicted prior to 1945. They offered seven explanations for the longevity of these chronic narcotics addicts. First, they felt that the long-lived patients may have a genetic advantage, since they often had parents living to an old age. Second, they were generally able to obtain a regular supply of narcotics, without having to survive withdrawal due to periods of abstinence. Third, these addicts had lifestyles which permitted them to avoid the violence which is common in the street narcotics subculture. Many were middle-level narcotics dealers, high-class prostitutes, or "businessmen" dealing in stolen merchandise. They lived by their wits and remained apart from persons who used violence to resolve disputes.

A fourth apparent reason for their longevity was their concern for cleaning the needles used for injecting narcotics. They were thus able to avoid the wide variety of dangerous infections which are transmitted by sharing needles. Fifth, they used alcohol and other drugs only moderately. Many other narcotics addicts are also addicted to alcohol or abuse other drugs which pose severe dangers to one's health.

A sixth reason for their longevity may be their "moderate" use of heroin. Most maintained a pattern of using enough heroin to avoid withdrawal symptoms, but avoided "binges," or overuse when the supply of the drug was easier to obtain.

The final possible reason for their longevity was their participation in methadone maintenance programs in recent years. Many had relied upon a physician for their supply of drugs earlier in life. Many of these physicians were older and either died or retired from practice. Since they were becoming too old to "hustle" drugs in the illicit street market, methadone maintenance programs offered a viable alternative which protected the older addicts from the dangers of the street drugs.

On the basis of existing research on heroin use, it seems likely that the number of older heroin addicts will increase in future years, as the younger generations of heroin addicts grow old. It does not seem that the use of heroin, *per se*, increases mortality when the drug is used in moderation and numerous precautions are taken. However, the illegal use of street heroin constitutes a great danger to the user due to the unreliability of the quality of the drugs and the dangers inherent in dealing with the street market.

Older persons seem to participate well in methadone maintenance programs in which methadone is prescribed as a substitute for heroin in the context of a community treatment program.

At the end of the last century, narcotic drugs were widely available from various legal sources. Today, narcotics are illegal, but still available in a dangerous street market where prices are high, violence is rampant and the quality of the drug is often questionable. Many of today's older narcotics addicts have maintained their drug habits despite many changes in society's attitudes and practices concerning the regulation of narcotic drugs. The experience of various drug treatment centres suggests that long-term addicts do not often give up their habits as the result of treatment. They are often fearful of the withdrawal process. However, older narcotics addicts often benefit from participation in methadone maintenance programs, where a legally prescribed drug is substituted for illegally obtained narcotics.

CONCLUSIONS

In this chapter we considered the prevention of problems associated with the use of different drugs by older persons. Very often, because of a biased attitude that it is "natural" to experience certain problems as one gets older, the possibility that many symptoms experienced by the elderly are drug-related is often overlooked. Problems related to the use of prescription medications, over-the-counter drugs and alcohol often appear in the form of confusion, tiredness, agitation or general feelings of discomfort which, according to common beliefs, one should expect as part of the natural processes of aging. For this reason, doctors may ignore danger signs, and older people and their relatives may put off seeking help until the problems become so severe that a crisis situation has developed.

One of the most important drug-associated problems is the adverse interactions between different medications, including alcohol. Research shows that older persons rarely receive appropriate information about drug interactions and are not often told how to recognize when they are having drug-related problems.

Who should be responsible for the prevention of drug-related problems in old age? In Canada, little emphasis has been placed upon the specific drug problems of older persons. Physicians receive relatively little training in the special aspects of prescribing for the elderly. Pharmacists do not systematically explain about the medications they dispense. Older persons themselves are not often aware of the effects, side effects, interactions, indications and contraindications of the medication they consume. All persons involved in the drug dispensing and selection network must be involved if more and better information is to be made available in order to help people make more sane choices about drug use.

It is obvious that without government intervention, changes in drug-related practices are not improving at a significant rate. For example, studies show that various aids to medication use, such as date-carded dispensing (where each pill is packaged on a card next to a clearly indicated date and time when the pill should be taken), greatly improve compliance with medication routines. Special information cards given out with all medications, including OTC drugs, increase awareness of dangerous interactions between drugs and possible negative side effects and help avoid many potential problems. Yet such relatively inexpensive aids are not widely available in Canada simply because no one is obligated to provide them. Perhaps it is time for the government to develop public policies for saner medication use in the elderly. Such prevention programs would probably be quite cost effective, since they would help avoid costly medical interventions due to improper use of drugs.

Besides the development of improvements in the communication of information about drugs and dispensing practices, attitudes need to be changed in order to assure that older persons with drug-related problems receive the help they need. Older alcoholics and heroin addicts are often refused treatment because of unfounded prejudices that older persons cannot benefit as much from therapeutic interventions, compared to younger age groups. Research to date has shown that this prejudice is unfounded. Older participants in various types of secondary and tertiary prevention programs for the treatment of alcoholism and heroin addiction have at least as good a chance of improving as younger participants. In fact, younger participants have a lower probability of profiting from treatments, according to several research reports. Thus, an improvement in the general attitude of caregivers towards older persons would serve to improve the quality of the services older persons receive as well as increase the chances that older persons with drug problems will receive the type of help they need.

Unfortunately, we have been forced to talk about older persons as if they constitute a homogeneous group with similar characteristics. We have done so because there are so few studies of individual differences in drug problems among the elderly that any discussion of individual differences would be sheer speculation. Individual differences clearly exist. In fact, research in gerontology suggests that individual differences in the elderly may be greater than individual differences in other age groups. One of the primary tasks for future research is to clarify the nature of individual differences in practices related to drug use in the elderly.

NOTES

1. Aminopyrine, Antipyrine, Dihydrostreptomycin and Sulfamethizole are not available in Canada.

CHAPTER 7

DRUGS AND THE ELDERLY: DIRECTIONS FOR PRACTICE, POLICY AND RESEARCH

Current research on age-related changes in drug effects indicate that there are clear differences which are related to age. In some instances, the differences reflect common changes which tend to occur as people grow older, but do not necessarily occur for all people. Some changes related to aging require corrective action to maintain youthful functioning. For example, the distribution and concentration of certain drugs are affected by the proportion of fatty body mass. If people do not modify their eating habits in middle age, their body fat increases due to changes in metabolism and digestion. Although older persons tend to be fatter, there are great individual differences. Being old does not necessarily mean being fatter. Some older persons have proportionately much less body fat than many younger people. Therefore, it is dangerous to overgeneralize from age differences which can be explained by changes in the proportion of body fat associated with normal aging. Average differences between older and younger persons may reflect culturally determined behaviour patterns, such as eating habits and the resulting differences in body fat, which may be changed by appropriate interventions (such as dieting).

Other changes, such as the increased likelihood of having chronic illnesses, may not be so easy to avoid. However, there are significant individual differences in health status in old age. Old people may, on the *average*, show significant differences from younger age groups. However, these differences may be avoidable (*e.g.*, by eating properly, dieting or exercising) and certainly do not affect all older people. They cannot be used to tell if any particular older person is different from any particular younger person.

Other age differences may be more universal, and may reflect more general processes which occur as part of the "natural" processes of aging. Some of these processes are not yet well understood. For example, there is research data suggesting that there are changes in sensitivity to benzodiazepines which are related to aging but independent of the pharmacokinetic properties of the drug.

One of the important tasks of future research is to differentiate between differences which are inherently linked to processes of aging and differences which are more likely to occur in older populations, but are not linked to general processes involved in growing older. For example, older persons are much more likely than younger persons to have chronic illnesses. Various illnesses can alter the effects of drugs. To date, most research simply compares older and younger populations and looks at significant differences between the averages for the two groups. More sophisticated research is needed in which people are not only classified according to their age, but concurrent differences, such as in the proportion of fatty tissue and presence of chronic diseases, are evaluated as possible explanations for the observed differences, independent of differences in chronological age.

Most research on drugs and older persons is cross-sectional in nature. In cross-sectional research older and younger persons are compared at one point in time. There is no way of knowing whether the differences observed are due to changes which occurred as people grew older, or if they simply reflect differences which exist between the current generation of older persons and the current generation of younger people. Perhaps, due to differences in upbringing, nutrition, etc., people who are now old are different from young people, but the older generation has not changed much since they were young. The only means of effectively evaluating if the age differences we observe reflect true changes with aging is to conduct longitudinal and sequential studies where the same persons are followed over time as they age. Longitudinal and sequential studies are costly and time consuming. However, without longitudinal data it is only a matter of faith that allows researchers to say that they are describing processes which are related to aging, rather than differences between different cohort groups of people born in different years.

Longitudinal research is not a panacea for all the problems involved in differentiating cohort differences from age change. Longitudinal studies may be influenced by changes which occur in society and the environment during the course of the study. For example, a longitudinal study of changes in attitudes towards drug use may reflect changes which are related to aging. However, they may just as well reflect changes in societal beliefs and practices which occurred during the course of the study. Longitudinal research has the inherent problem of confounding age changes with external changes which occur for all people during the course of the study.[1]

The chapter on the restoration and preservation of youth leaves one disappointed by the fact that to date we have no miracle drugs to prolong youth and retard the aging processes. Seekers of such miraculous products are probably doomed from the start in their quests. Aging involves many concurrent processes which occur at different levels, at different rates and have multiple causes. Since there is probably no single cause of aging, it would be futile to seek a single substance which would reverse or inhibit aging. While successful immortalist interventions are unlikely, we can probably hope for the development of new and better drugs to help with the many diseases and problems which occur more frequently in old age.

As we have seen, having effective drugs can be useless or even harmful if they are not prescribed with wisdom and taken with care. Along with the drugs we need to develop better systems to ensure proper use. As we indicated in Chapter 4, perhaps the most effective means of maintaining youth and prolonging life are not drugs at all. Changing one's eating habits and exercising regularly are among the most promising interventions known to date. Perhaps what is really needed is the development of non-pharmacological interventions. It may very well be that, because of their potential dangers, drugs should be held in reserve in the battle against the problems associated with old age.

Drugs are not good or evil. All drugs can be dangerous if abused. Many of the most feared drugs in our society pose relatively few dangers when used properly. Other seemingly harmless substances can have deadly results when abused. For example, aspirin is one of the major drugs responsible for overdose deaths in Canada. On the other hand, research shows that heroin addicts who observe certain precautions can live to a ripe old age in good health despite a lifetime of use of this illegal drug. Alcohol may have beneficial effects when consumed in moderation. However, alcohol abuse is one of the surest means of increasing the probability of a premature death. Problems which arise from drug use are mostly due to the patterns of use rather than the inherent "bad" nature of the substances themselves.

Still, the Canadian government classifies drugs as good ("approved for use" with or without prescription) and bad ("illegal" and "dangerous"). Much government money is spent on enforcing these distinctions. Far less money is spent on assuring that drugs are used in a proper manner. Several aids to appropriate drug use were proposed in the chapter on prevention. It is hoped that some day the appropriate agencies will take a closer look at how drug-related problems can be prevented and institute some of the fairly simple and cost effective programs for the elderly reviewed in this book. For example, it is possible that a law requiring all pharmacists to give elderly prescription drug users a special "geriatric" version of the Supplementary Information on Medication sheets developed by the Canadian Pharmaceutical Association whenever they fill a prescription may help avoid much drug misuse and help older consumers become more aware of signs of dangerous side effects and drug interactions.

Older persons who have drug-related problems often do not receive appropriate help. This is due to problems in diagnosis and prejudices about the benefits of treatment for older people. Drug problems are often not diagnosed because of the belief that symptoms are "natural" parts of growing old, rather than reflective of problems which may be alleviated. Despite research results to the contrary, practitioners continue to deny older persons treatment because they erroneously feel that older people do not benefit as much from interventions. In order to develop effective drug prevention programs we must educate practitioners and older persons themselves to recognize possible danger signs and to utilize available methods and resources for obtaining help with drug-related problems.

For certain types of drug-related problems, older persons may have fewer problems than younger age groups. For example, research indicates that significant numbers of older persons reduce their consumption of alcohol and cigarettes in the later years of life. Perhaps if we were better able to understand the mechanisms involved in such voluntary changes resulting in "saner" drug use, we would learn how to more effectively help younger persons avoid and reduce drug-related problems.

In this book we have discussed older persons as if they constituted a clearly identifiable group with similar characteristics. As we have pointed out, there are great individual differences in all aspects of drug effects and drug use in the elderly. Quite clearly, it is this increased variability and lack of predictability that makes prescribing for the elderly such a complex task for physicians. Unfortunately, little research has been conducted to clarify the nature of important dimensions of individual differences. There are few studies on ethnic and cultural differences among the elderly and their influences on drug use and abuse. The subject of individual differences and their determinants is probably where the most research needs to be conducted. Perhaps if researchers begin to see older persons more as individuals than just as members of a homogeneous group, research on drugs and older people will move a giant step closer to helping understand the true nature of drug use and abuse in the everday lives of older Canadians.

NOTES

1. For a more detailed discussion of the relative advantages and disadvantages of different research methodologies for studying aging see Mishara and Riedel 1984.

GLOSSARY

Absorption The process by which a drug moves from outside the body to its site of action.

Achlorhydria An age-related condition where the acidity of the stomach is reduced.

Aerobic exercise Exercise that improves the ability of the heart and lungs to carry oxygen to the body.

Aging There are many aspects of aging, biological, social, emotional, so that describing a person's age in years (chronological age) is usually inadequate. Unfortunately, most research into aging defines "elderly" as over 65. This is because chronological age is easy to measure, and generally accepted measures of other types of aging have not been developed.

Ataxia A decrease in movement or a loss in the ability to move.

Benzodiazepines A class of drugs used to induce sleep and reduce anxiety. Librium and Valium belong to this class.

Chi-square test A statistical test of categorical data that determines the likelihood that a group or groups are drawn from a specific population.

Cohort effect In cross-sectional studies groups of different ages are compared. Differences between these groups may be due to differences in age, but they may also be due to the fact that people of different ages grew up in different circumstances. This latter source of differences between people of different ages is called the "cohort effect" and should not be considered an effect of aging as such.

Compliance The extent to which a patient complies with or adheres to the instructions of a physician.

Contraindication A sign, symptom or other indication that a drug should not be prescribed or consumed.

Cross-tolerance When tolerance that has developed to the repeated administration of one drug causes a diminished response to a different drug.

DAR Drug Adverse Reaction. Any effect of a drug not wanted by the physician or the patient.

Dependence The repeated and reliable self-administration of a drug.

Distribution The description of how a drug is spread to different parts of the body.

Drug   A substance, usually refined, that interacts with the physiology of the body. Normally, foods and substances taken for nourishment are excluded from such a definition.

Elderly   See aging.

Elimination   The process whereby drugs are removed from the body.

Enzyme   A catalyst of a chemical reaction. Enzymes control the chemical reactions in the body.

Excipient   A substance added to an active ingredient in a medicine. These additives may be used for such purposes as dilution, binding, lubrication colouring and flavouring. They are supposed to be inert, but this is not always the case.

Free radicals   Molecules with an unpaired electron. Free radicals can combine with molecules in body cells and damage them. Such a process has been proposed by some researchers to account for aging.

Generic name   A universally agreed-upon name referring to a particular chemical which may be marketed under a variety of trade names. The generic name is usually used in text books and scientific writing.

Immortalist interventions   An approach to the treatment of aging that seeks to prolong the absolute lifespan by altering the basic processes of aging.

Incrementalist interventions   Approach to the treatment of aging by seeking to avoid accidents and diseases of old age, but not necessarily prolonging the pro-grammed age.

McCay effect   In 1936 McCay found that restricted diet would prolong the life expectancy of rats. This effect has been replicated many times and is believed to apply to humans.

Maturing out   The idea that many drug users spontaneously reduce or stop using a drug as they mature or get older.

Meliorist interventions   This approach to the treatment of aging seeks to reduce the impact of aging and the diseases of aging by reducing their symptoms and improv-ing the quality of life of elderly people.

Metabolism   The process of changing the structure of molecules by the chemistry of the body.

Methylxanthines   The family of drugs to which caffeine belongs. They are also known as the xanthine stimulants. Other members of the family are theophylline found in tea and theobromine found in chocolate.

Nephron   The functional unit of the kidney.

OTC   Over-The-Counter (medicine). A medicine that is available without a prescription from a physician.

Pharmacokinetics   This term refers to the movement of drugs into the body to the site of action and then out of the body.

Physical dependence   After a drug has been taken for some time, withdrawal symptoms will occur when the drug is discontinued.

Polypharmacy   The prescribing (or consumption of) several different drugs at the same time by the same person.

Primary prevention   Measures aimed at preventing or inhibiting the development of problems before they begin.

Psychological dependence   This term is not useful because the terms "dependence" and "physical dependence" can account for all phenomena. It is used by some authors to explain drug use in the absence of physical dependence, but this is only necessary if one assumes that withdrawal symptoms are the only motivation to use drugs. There is little evidence that this is so.

Regression analysis   A complex statistical procedure where many different variables (predictor variables) are correlated with another variable (dependent variable). Regression analysis is used to determine the extent to which each of the predictor variables can independently account for individual differences in the independent variable.

Secondary prevention   Measures aimed at reducing the prevalence of a problem.

Shunamatism   The ancient practice of sleeping with a younger person for the sake of absorbing some vital spirit of youth.

Site of action   The place (or places) in the body where a drug causes its effect. Drugs that do not reach their site of action have no effect.

Tertiary prevention   Measures aimed at reducing the impact of a problem rather than preventing it's occurrence or spread.

Therapeutic index   The relative safety of a drug, described frequently as the ratio of an effective dose of a drug to a dose that causes adverse reactions or death.

Trade name   The name given to the specific formulation of a generic drug by a manufacturer.

Withdrawal symptoms   Physiological changes that occur when drug is withdrawn from a physically dependent person.

BIBLIOGRAPHY

Addiction Research Foundation
1984   *Statistics on Alcohol and Drug Use in Canada and other Countries* (Vol. 2). *Statistics on Drug Use.* Toronto: Addiction Research Foundation.
1985a   *Facts About Alcohol.* Toronto: Alcoholism and Drug Addiction Research Foundation.
1985b   *Cannabis.* Toronto: Addiction Research Foundation.
Adelman, C.
1985   "Biological Aging: Theories and Current Research." Paper Presented at the Annual Meeting of the *Canadian Association on Gerontology:* Hamilton.
Advisory Committee on the Management of Severe Chronic Pain in Cancer Patients
1984   *Cancer Pain.* Ottawa: Minister of Supply and Services Canada (Catalogue No. H42-214).
American Association of Retired Persons
1984   *Prescription Drugs: A Survey of Consumer Use, Attitudes and Behavior.* Washington, D.C.
Anderson, A. J., J. J. Barboriak, and A. A. Rimm
1978   "Risk Factors and Angiographically Determined Coronary Occlusion." *American Journal of Epidemiology* 107:8–14.
Atkinson, L., I. I. J. M. Gibson, and J. Andrews
1977   "The Difficulties of Old People Taking Drugs." *Age and Aging* 6:144–50.
1978   "An Investigation into the Ability of Elderly Patients Continuing to Take Prescribed Drugs after Discharge from Hospital and Recommendations Concerning Improving the Situation." *Gerontology* 24:225–34.
Baker, W. W.
1985   "Pharmacology of Aging: Use, Misuse, and Abuse of Psychotropic Drugs." In E. Gottheil, K. A. Druley, T. E. Skoloda and H. M. Waxman (eds.), *The Combined Problems of Alcoholism, Drug Addiction and Aging.* Springfield, Illinois: Charles C. Thomas.
Barone, J. J., and H. Roberts
1984   "Human Consumption of Caffeine." In P. B. Dews (ed.), *Caffeine Perspectives from Recent Research.* Berlin: Springer-Verlag.
Barrows, C. H., and R. E. Beauchene
1970   "Aging and Nutrition." In A. A. Albanese (ed.), *Newer Methods of Nutritional Biochemistry* (Vol. 4). New York: Academic Press.

Bates, T. R., J. M. Young, L. M. Wu, and H. A. Rosenberg
  1974   "A pH-dependent Dissolution Rate of Nitrofurantion from Commercial
         Suspensions, Tablets and Capsules." *Journal of Pharmaceutical Science*
         63:643.

Belloc, N.
  1973   "Relationship of Health Practices and Mortality." *Preventive Medicine*
         2:67–81.

Benet, L. Z., A. Greither, and W. Meister
  1976   "Gastrointestinal Absorption of Drugs in Patients with Cardiac
         Failure." In L. Z. Benet (ed.), *The Effect of Disease States on Pharma-
         cokinetics*. Washington, D.C.: American Pharmaceutical Association.

Bennion, L., and T. K. Li
  1976   "Alcohol Metabolism in American Indians and Whites." *The New
         England Journal of Medicine* 194:9–13.

Bernstein, A., and H. L. Lennard
  1973   "Drugs, Doctors and Junkies." *Society* 10:14–25.

Blackwell, B.
  1979   "Drug Regimes and Treatment Compliance." In R. B. Hayes, D. W.
         Taylor and D. L. Sackett (eds.), *Compliance and Health Care*.
         Baltimore: The Johns Hopkins University Press.

Blaney, R., I. S. Radford, and G. A. MacKenzie
  1975   "Belfast Study of the Prediction of Outcome of Alcoholism." *British
         Journal of Addiction* 70:41–50.

Block, L.
  1982   "Polymedicine: Known and Unknown Drug Interactions." *Journal of
         the American Geriatrics Society* 30:S94–S98.

Bosse, R., A. J. Garvey, and R. J. Glynn
  1980   "Age and Addiction to Smoking." *Addictive Behaviors* 5:341–51.

Bourne, P. G.
  1973   "Drug Abuse in the Aging." *Perspectives on Aging* 2:18–20.

Brand, F. N., R. T. Smith, P. A. Brand
  1977   "Effects of Economic Barriers to Medical Care on Patients' Non-
         compliance." *Public Health Reports* 92:72–78.

Bressler, R.
  1982   "Adverse Drug Reactions." In K. A. Conrad and R. Bressler (eds.),
         Drug Therapy for the Elderly. St. Louis: The C. V. Mosby Company,
         64–85.

Butler, R. N.
  1975   *Why Survive? Growing Old in America*. New York: Harper & Row.
  1985   "Senile Dementia: Reversible and Irreversible." *The Counseling
         Psychologist* 12(2):75–79.

Canada Health Survey
  1981   *The Health of Canadians*. Report of the Canada Health Survey.
         (Catalogue No. 82-538E). Ottawa: Ministry of Supply and Services.

Canadian Foundation on Alcohol and Drug Dependencies
  1977   "Alcohol and Drug Problems among the Native Peoples of Canada."
         Communications 3:2–11.

Cape, R. D. T.
    1979   "Drugs and Confusion States." In J. Crooks and I. H. Stevenson (eds.),
    Drugs and the Elderly: Perspectives in Geriatric and Clinical Pharmacology. Baltimore: University Park Press 267–77.

Capel, W., and L. Peppers
    1978   "The Aging Addict: A Longitudinal Study of Known Abusers." *Addictive Diseases: An International Journal*, 3:389–403.

Caranasos, G. J., G. B. Stewart, and L. E. Cluff
    1974   "Drug-induced Illness Leading to Hospitalization." *Journal of the American Medical Association* 228:713–17.

Carruth, B.
    1973   "Toward a Definition of Problem Drinking among Older Persons: Conceptual and Methodological Considerations." In E. P. Williams *et al.* (eds.), *Alcohol and Problem Drinking Among Older Persons*. Springfield, Virginia: National Technical Information Service.

Chambers, C. D., O. Z. White, and J. H. Lindquist
    1983   "Physician Attitudes and Prescribing Practices." *Journal of Psychoactive Drugs* 15(1–2):55–59.

Charney, E.
    1975   "Compliance and Prescribance." *American Journal of Diseases of Children* 129:1009–1010.

Chien, C., E. Townsend, and A. Townsend
    1978   "Substance Use and Abuse Among the Community Elderly: The Medical Aspect." *Addictive Diseases: An International Journal* 3:357–72.

Clairmont, D.
    1963   *Deviance Among Indians and Eskimos in Aklavik, N.W.T.* Ottawa: Department of Northern Affairs and National Resources.

Cohen, S., and K. Ditman
    1973   "Gerovital H3 in the Treatment of the Depressed Aging Patient." *Psychosomatics* 15:15–19.

Colditz, G. A., G. L. Branch, R. J. Lipnick, W. C. Willett, B. Rosner, B. Posner, and C. H. Hennekens
    1985   "Moderate Alcohol and Decreased Cardiovascular Mortality in the Elderly Cohort." *American Heart Journal* 109(4):886–89.

Comfort, A.
    1973   "Effects of Ethoxyquin in the Longevity of C3H Mice." *Nature* 229:254–55.

Cooper, J. K., D. W. Love, and P. R. Raffoul
    1984   "Intentional Prescription Nonadherence (Noncompliance) by the Elderly." *Journal of the American Geriatrics Society* 30(5):329–33.

Cupit, G.
    1982   "The Use of Non-Prescription Analgesics in an Older Population." *Journal of the American Geriatrics Society* 30:S76–S80.

Curley, R. T.
    1967   "Drinking Patterns of the Mescalero Apache." *Quarterly Journal of Studies on Alcohol* 28:116–31.

Das, B. C.
  1977   "Drug Taking is a Serious Business for the Old." *Modern Geriatrics* 7:22–23.
Data Laboratories
  1978   *Report of a Survey of Canadian Attitudes Towards Smoking*. Unpublished report.
Davidson, W.
  1979   "Drugs for Eternal Youth: Scientific Attempts to Combat Aging." *Journal of Drug Issues* 9(1):91–104.
  1985   "Adverse Drug Reactions in the Elderly." In R. N. Butler and A. G. Bearn (eds.), *The Aging Process: Therapeutic Implications*. New York: Raven Press, 101–16.
de Beauvoir, S.
  1972   *The Coming of Age*. New York: G. P. Putnam's and Sons.
Department of National Health and Welfare, Bureau of Dangerous Drugs, Health Protection Branch
  1984   *Drug Users and Convictions Statistics 1977, 1978, 1979, and 1981 and Narcotic, Controlled and Restricted Drug Statistics 1982*. Ottawa: Department of National Health and Welfare, undated. As reported in Addiction Research Foundation.
DesJarlais, D. C., H. Joseph, and D. T. Courtwright
  1985   "Old Age and Addiction: A Study of Elderly Patients in Methadone Maintenance Treatment." In E. Gottheil, K. A. Druley, T. E. Skoloda and H. M. Waxman (eds.). *The Combined Problems of Alcoholism, Drug Addiction and Aging*. Springfield, Illinois: Charles C. Thomas, 201–209.
DHEW
  1979   *The Aging Process and Psychoactive Drug Use*. Washington, D.C.: Government Printing Office.
Dozier, E. P.
  1966   "Problem Drinking Among American Indians: The Role of Sociocultural Deprivation." *Quarterly Journal of Studies on Alcohol* 27:72–87.
Drestren, H.
  1961   "Essai Clinique de la Centrophenoxine en Gériatrie." *La Presse Médicale* 69:1999–2001.
Drew, L. R. H.
  1968   "Alcohol as a Self-limiting Disease." *Quarterly Journal of Studies on Alcoholism* 29:956–67.
Drori, D., and Folman, Y.
  1971   "The Effect of Mating on the Longevity of Male Rats." *Experimental Gerontology* 14:363–66.
Dunker, T., and R. Tippit
  1973   *Live Longer Through Sex*. Hermosa Beach, California: Concord House.
Eckardt, M. J., T. C. Harford, C. T. Koelber, E. S. Parker, L. S. Rosenthal, R. S. Ryback, G. C. Salmoiraghi, E. Vamderveen, and D. R. Warren
  1981   "Health Hazards Associated with Alcohol Consumption." *Journal of the American Medical Association* 246:658–66.

Elsayed, M., A. H. Isamaiel, and R. J. Young
  1980   "Intellectual Differences of Adult Men Related to Age and Physical Fitness Before and After an Exercise Program." *Journal of Gerontology* 35:383–87.

Ettlinger, P. R. A., and G. K. Freeman
  1981   "General Practice Compliance Study: Is it Worth Being a Personal Doctor?" *British Medical Journal* 282:1192–94.

Evans, J. G., and E. H. Jarvis
  1972   "Nitrazepam and the Elderly." *British Medical Journal* 5838:487.

Eve, S. E., and H. J. Friedsam
  1981   "Use of Tranquilizers and Sleeping Pills among Older Texans." *Journal of Psychoactive Drugs* 13(1–2):165–73.

Farkas, C. S.
  1979   "Caffeine Intake and Potential Effect on Health of a Segment of North Canadian Indigenous People." *International Journal of Addictions* 14:27–32.

Fedder, D.
  1982   "Managing Medication and Compliance: Physician-Pharmacist-Patient Interactions." *Journal of the American Geriatrics Society* 30:S113–S117.

Forbes, G. B., and J. C. Reina
  1970   "Adult Lean Body Mass Declines with Age, Some Longitudinal Observations." *Metabolism* 19:653.

Foster, D., L. Klinger-Vartabedain, and L. Wispe
  1984   "Male Longevity and Age Differences Between Spouses." *Journal of Gerontology* 39(1):117–20.

Gambert, S. R., M. Newton, and E. H. Duthie
  1984   "Medical Issues in Alcoholism in the Elderly." In J. T. Hartford and T. Samorajski (eds.). *Alcoholism in the Elderly: Social and Biomedical Issues*. New York: Raven Press, 174–92.

Gerbino, P., and J. Gans
  1982   "Antacids and Laxatives for Symptomatic Relief in the Elderly." *Journal of the American Geriatrics Society* 30:S81–S87.

German, S., L. E. Klein, S. J. McPhee, and C. R. Smith
  1984   "Knowledge of and Compliance with Drug Regimes in the Elderly." *Journal of the American Geriatrics Society* 30(9):568–71.

Gilbert, R. M.
  1976   "Caffeine as a Drug of Abuse." In R. J. Gibbins, Y. Israel, H. Kalant, R. E. Popham, W. Schmidt and R. G. Smart (eds.). *Research Advances in Alcohol and Drug Problems*. New York: Wiley.
  1984   "Caffeine Consumption." In A. Spiller (ed.). *The Methylxanthine Beverages and Foods: Chemistry, Consumption, and Health Effects*. New York: Alan R. Liss, 185–213.

Gilbert, R. M., J. A. Marshman, M. Schweider, and R. Berg
  1976   "Caffeine Content of Beverages as Consumed." *Canadian Medical Association Journal* 114:205–211.

Glantz, M.
  1981   "Predictions of Elderly Drug Abuse." *Journal of Psychoactive Drugs* 13(2):117–26.

Glazer, G. B., and Zawadski, R. T.
    1981   "Use of Psychotropic Drugs Among the Aged Revisited." *Journal of Psychoactive Drugs* 13(2):195–98.

Greenblatt, D. J.
    1979   "Reduced Serum Albumen Concentration in the Elderly: A Report from the Boston Collaborative Drug Surveillance Program." *Journal of the American Geriatrics Society* 27:20.

Greenblatt, D. J., M. Allen, and R. I. Shader
    1977   "Toxicity of High Dose Flurazepam in the Elderly." *Clinical Pharmacology and Therapeutics* 21:355–61.

Greenblatt, D. J., E. B. Sellers, and R. I. Shader
    1982   "Drug Disposition in Old Age." *New England Journal of Medicine* 306(18):1081–88.

Greiner, R., I. Bross, and H. Gold
    1974   "A Method of Evaluation of Laxative Habits in Human Subjects." *Journal of Chronic Diseases* 6:244–52.

Grove, W. R., and M. Hughes
    1979   "Possible Causes of Apparent Sex Differences in Physical Health: An Empirical Investigation." *American Sociological Review* 44:126–46.

Gruner, O. C.
    1930   *A Treatise on the Canon of Medicine of Avicenna.* London: Luzac.

Guttman, D.
    1978   "Patterns of Legal Drug Use by Older Americans." *Addictive Diseases* 3:337–56.

Hall, M. R. P.
    1973   "Drug Therapy in the Elderly." *British Medical Journal* 4:582–94.

Hammel, R. W., and P. O. Williams
    1964   "Do Patients Receive Prescribed Medication?" *Journal of the American Pharmaceutical Association* 4:331–37.

Hanlon, V.
    1979   *The Clinical Significance of Non-compliance among the Elderly: A Report on Problems and Considerations.* Summer Resources Funds Project No. 1216-8-50, Health Promotion Directorate, Health and Welfare Canada.

Harman, D.
    1968   "Free Radical Theory of Aging: Effects of Free Radical Reaction Inhibitors on the Mortality Rate of the Male LAF_1 Mice." *Journal of Gerontology* 23:476–82.

Haynes, R. B.
    1976   "A Critical Review of the 'Determinants' of Patient Compliance with Therapeutic Regimes." In D. L. Sackett and R. B. Haynes (eds.). *Compliance with Therapeutic Regimes.* Baltimore: Johns Hopkins University Press, 26–39.

Haynes, R. B., D. L. Sackett, D. W. Taylor, R. S. Roberts, and A. L. Johnson
    1977   "Manipulation of the Therapeutic Regime to Improve Compliance: Conceptions and Misconceptions." *Clinical Pharmacology and Therapeutics* 22(2):125–30.

Health Protection Branch
    1985   "Heroin." *Information Letter*, 699(6). Ottawa: Health and Welfare Canada.

Helzer, J. E., K. E. Carey, and R. H. Miller
    1984   "Predictors and Correlates of Recovery in Older versus Younger Alcoholics." In G. Maddox, L. N. Robbins and N. Rosenberg (eds.). *Nature and Extent of Alcohol Problems Among the Elderly*. Rockville, Maryland: U.S. Department of Health and Human Services, 83–99. (National Institute of Alcohol Abuse and Alcoholism, Research Monograph No. 14).

Hulka, B. S.
    1979   "Patient-clinician Interactions and Compliance." In R. B. Haynes, D. W. Taylor, and D. L. Sachett (eds.), *Compliance and Health Care*. Baltimore: The Johns Hopkins University Press, 63–77.

Hurd, P. D., and J. Blevins
    1984   "Aging and the Color of Pills." *New England Journal of Medicine* 310(3), 202.

Hurwitz, N.
    1969   "Predisposing Factors in Adverse Reactions to Drugs." *British Medical Journal* 1:536–639.

Inciardi, J. A., D. C. Bride, B. R. Russe, and K. S. Wells
    1978   "Acute Drug Reactions Among the Aged: A Research Note." *Addictive Diseases: An International Journal* 3(3):383–88.

Indian and Northern Affairs Canada
    1980   *Indian Conditions: A Survey*. Ottawa: Indian and Northern Affairs Canada.

Kastenbaum, R.
    1972   "Beer, Wine and Mutual Gratification in the Gerontopolis." In D. P. Kent, S. Sherwood, and R. Kastenbaum (eds.). *Research, Action and Planning for the Elderly*. New York: Behavioral Publications, 37–49.

Kastenbaum, R., and Slater
    1972   "Effects of Wine on the Interpersonal Behavior of Geriatric Patients: An Exploratory Study." In R. Kastenbaum (ed.), *New Thoughts on Old Age*. New York: Springer, 191-204.

Kiernan, P. J., and J. B. Issacs
    1981   "Use of Drugs by the Elderly." *Journal of the Royal Society of Medicine* 74:196–200.

Klatsky, A. L., G. D. Friedman, and A. B. Siegelaub
    1974   "Alcohol Consumption before Myocardial Infarction: Results from the Kaiser-Permanente Epidemiological Study on Myocardial Infarction." *Annals of Internal Medicine* 81:294–301.

Klein, M. D., P. S. German, D. M. Levine, E. R. Feroli, and J. Ardery
    1984   "Medication Problems among Outpatients. A study with Emphasis on the Elderly." *Archives of Internal Medicine* 144:1185–88.

Kofoed, L. L.
    1984   "Abuse and Misuse of Over-the-Counter Drugs by Elderly." In R. M.

Atkinson (ed.). *Alcohol and Drug Abuse in Old Age.* Washington: American Psychiatric Press, 50–59.

Kohn, R. R.
1971   "Effects of Anti-oxidants on Life Span of C57BL Mice." *Journal of Gerontology* 26:378–80.

Kurtzman, J., and P. Gordon
1976   *No More Dying.* Los Angeles: J. P. Tarcher.

Lampe, K. F.
1985   "Physician Instructions to the Patient." In S. R. Moore and T. W. Teal (eds.). *Geriatric Drug Use: Clinical and Social Perspectives.* New York: Pergamon press, 34–38.

Lamy, P. P.
1978   "Therapeutics and the Elderly." *Addictive Diseases: An International Journal,* 3:311–55.

1981   "Drug Prescribing for the Elderly." *Bulletin of the New York Academy of Medicine* 57:718–30.

1982   "Comparative Pharmacokinetic Changes and Drug Therapy in the Older Population," *Journal of the American Geriatrics Society* 30:S11–S19.

1982   "Over the Counter Medication: The Drug Interactions We Overlook." *Journal of the American Geriatrics Society* 30:S69–S74.

1985   "The Aging: Drug Use and Misuse." In E. Gottheil, K. A. Druley, T. E. Skoloda and H. M. Waxman (eds.). *The Combined Problems of Alcoholism, Drug Addiction and Aging.* Springfield, Illinois: Charles C. Thomas, 130–49.

1985   "Patterns of Prescribing and Drug Use." In R. N. Butler and A. G. Bearn (eds.). *The Aging Process: Therapeutic Implication.* New York: Raven Press

Laties, V., and B. Weiss
1962   "Behavioral Mechanisms of Drug Action." In P. Black (ed.). *Drugs and the Brain.* Baltimore: Johns Hopkins.

Law, R., and C. Chalmers
1976   "Medicines and Elderly People." *British Medical Journal* 1:565–68.

Leaf, A.
1973   *Life and Death and Medicine.* San Francisco: W. H. Freeman.

Learoyd, R. F.
1972   "Psychotropic Drugs and the Elderly Patient." *Medical Journal of Australia,* 1:1131–33.

Ledwidge, B.
1980   "Run for your Mind." *Canadian Journal of Behavioral Sciences* 12:126–40.

Leibovitz, B. E., and B. J. Siegel
1980   "Aspects of Free Radical Reactions: Aging." *Journal of Gerontology* 35(1):45–55.

Lemert, E. M.
1954   "Alcohol and the Northwest Coast Indians." University of California, *Publications in Culture and Society* 2:303–406.

1958 "The Use of Alcohol in Three Salish Indian Tribes." *Quarterly Journal for Studies in Alcohol,* 19:90–107.

Levy, G
1967 "Effect of Bed Rest on Distribution and Elimination of Drugs." *Journal of Pharmaceutical Science* 56:928.

Ley, P.
1979 "Memory for Medical Information." *British Journal of Social and Clinical Psychology* 19:311–16.

Linn, M.
1978 "Attrition of Older Alcoholics from Treatment." *Addictive Diseases: An International Journal* 3:437–47.

Little, A. G., and E. Withington
1928 *Di retardatione accidentium senctutis.* Oxford: Clarendon Press.

Lorand, A.
1911 *Old Age Deferred.* Philadelphia: F. A. Davis.

MacDonald, J. B., and E. T. MacDonald
1977 "Nocturnal Femoral Fractures and Continuing Widespread Use of Barbiturate Hypnotics." *British Medical Journal* 2:483–85.

Mallet, L., and M. Gervais
1984 "Implications of Pharmacists on a Geriatric Ward." Paper presented to the Canadian Association on Gerontology, Vancouver, *Program and Abstracts* 1:26.

Mandolini, A.
1981 "The Social Contexts of Aging and Drug Use: Theoretical and Methodological Insights." *Journal of Psychoactive Drugs* 13(2):135–42.

Marcus, A. C., and T. Seeman
1981 "Sex Differences in Health Status: A Re-examination of the Nurturant Role Hypothesis. (Comment on Grove and Hughes, 1979)." *American Sociological Review* 46:119–23.

Marmot, M. G., G. Rose, M. J. Shipley, and B. J. Thomas
1981 "Alcohol and Mortality: U-Shaped Curve." *Lancet* 1:580.

Martys, C. R.
1982 "Drug Treatments in Elderly Patients." *British Medical Journal* 283:1623–25.

Masoro, E. J., B. P. Yu, H. A. Bertrand, and F. T. Lynd
1980 "Nutritional Probe of the Aging Process." *Federation Proceedings* 39:3178–82.

May, F. E., R. B. Stewart, and L. E. Cluff
1977 "Drug Interactions and Multiple Drug Administrations." *Clinical Pharmacology and Therapeutics* 22:322.

May, F. E., R. B. Stewart, W. E. Hale, and R. E. Marks
1982 "Prescribed and Nonprescribed Drug Use in an Ambulatory Population." *Southern Medical Journal* 75:522–28.

Mayersohn, M
1982 "Drug Disposition." In K. A. Conrad and R. Bressler (eds.). *Drug Therapy for The Elderly.* St. Louis: C. V. Mosby Co.

McCay, C. M. and L. A. Maynard
1935 "Effects of Retarded Growth on the Length of Lifespan and upon the Ultimate Body Size." *Journal of Nutrition*, 10:63–79.

McCay, C. M., F. Pope, and W. Lunsford
1956 "Experimental Prolongation of Life Span." *Bulletin of the New York Academy of Medicine* 32:91–101.

McGlone, F. B., and E. Glick
1978 "Health Habits in Relation to Aging." *Journal of the American Geriatrics Society* 26(11):481–88.

McKim, W. A.
1986 *Drugs and Behavior, An Introduction to Behavioral Pharmacology.* Englewood Cliffs, New Jersey: Prentice-Hall.

McKim, W. A., M. J. Stones, and A. Kozma
1986 "Factors predicting medicine use in an elderly population." Paper presented at the annual meeting of the *Canadian Association on Gerontology*, Quebec City, 1986.

McPherson, B., and C. Kozlick
1980 "Canadian Leisure Patterns by Age: Disengagement, Continuity or Ageism." In V. W. Marshall (ed.). *Aging in Canada*. Don Mills: Fitzhenry and Whiteside.

Melmon, K. L.
1971 "Preventable Drug Reactions. Causes and Cures." *New England Journal of Medicine* 284(24):1361–68.

Millar, W. J.
1983 *Smoking Behavior of Canadians*. Ottawa: Ministry of Supply and Services Canada.

Mishara, B. L.
1985 "What We Know, Don't Know and Need to Know about Older Alcoholics." In E. Gottheil, K. A. Druley, T. E. Skoloda and H. M. Waxman (eds.). *The Combined Problems of Alcoholism, Drug Addiction and Aging.* Springfield, Illinois: Charles C. Thomas, 243–61.

Mishara, B. L., and R. Kastenbaum
1974 "Wine in the Treatment of Long-term Geriatric Patients in Mental Institutions." *Journal of the American Geriatrics Society* 22:88–94.
1980 *Alcohol and Old Age*. New York: Grune and Stratton.

Mishara, B. L., R. Kastenbaum, R. F. Baker, and R. Patterson
1975 "Alcohol Effects in Old Age: An Experimental Investigation." *Social Science and Medicine* 9:535–47.

Mishara, B. L., and R. Riedel
1984 *Le Vieillissement*. Paris: Presses Universitaires de France.

Mishara, B. L., and M. Wexler
1986 *Drug Use Among the Independent Elderly in Montreal*. Montreal: Unpublished Report, in preparation.

Mock, B.
1977 Rehabilitation of the Elderly Cardiac Patient Hampered by Bias. *Geriatrics* 32:22–23.

Moran, M. G. and T. L. Thompson, II
  1982   "Increased Psychotropic Side Effects in Geriatric Patients." *Hospital Formulary*, 17:1513–21.
Morgan, R. F.
  1981   *Interventions in Applied Gerontology*. Dubuque, Iowa: Kendall/Hunt Publishing Company.
Mosher, B. A.
  1982   *The Health Effects of Caffeine*. New York: American Council of Science of Health.
Murray, D.
  1974   *Multiple Drug Use Among the Elderly*. Faculty of Medicine, University of Manitoba, unpublished.
Musto, D., and M. Ramos
  1982   "Notes on American History: A Follow-up Study of the New Haven Morphine Maintenance Clinic of 1920." *New England Journal of Medicine* 304:1071–77.
Napke, E.
  1975   "Excipients and Additives: Hidden Hazards in Drug Products and in Product Substitution." *Canadian Medical Association Journal* 131:1449.
  1983   "Adverse Reactions: Some Pitfalls and Postulates." In M. N. G. Dukes (ed.), *Side Effects of Drugs. Annual 7*. Amsterdam: Excerpta Medica.
Nathanson, C. A.
  1975   "Illness and the Feminine Role: A Theoretical Review. *Social Science and Medicine* 11:13–25.
  1977   "Sex, Illness and Medical Care: A Review of Data, Theory and Method." *Social Science and Medicine* 11:13–25.
Neely, E., and M. L. Patrick
  1968   "Problems of Aged Persons Taking Medications at Home." *Nursing Research* 17:52–55.
O'Donnell, J. A.
  1969   *Narcotic Addicts in Kentucky*. Washinton, D.C.: Public Health Service Publications, No. 1881.
Olins, N. L.
  1985   "Pharmacy Interventions." In S. R. Moore and T. W. Teal (eds.). *Geriatric Drug Use: Clinical and Social Perspectives*. New York: Pergamon Press, 22–23.
Olson, J., and J. Johnson
  1977   "Drug Misuse Among the Elderly." *Journal of Gerontological Nursing* 4:11–14.
Parker, J., and H. Gerjuoy
  1979   "Life-span Extension: The State of the Art." In R. M. Veach (ed.). *Life Span: Values and Life Extending Technology*. San Francisco: Harper & Row.
Parkin, D. M., C. R. Henney, J. Quirk, and J. Crooks
  1976   "Deviation from Prescribed Drug Treatment After Discharge from Hospital." *British Medical Journal* 2:686–88.

Parry, H., M. Balter, and I. Cisin
    1971   "Primary Levels of Underreporting Psychotropic Drug Use." *Public Opinion Quarterly* 34:582–92.

Pascarelli, E. F., and W. Fischer
    1974   "Drug Dependence in the Elderly." *International Journal of Aging and Human Development* 5(4):347–56.

Peterson, D. M., F. J. Whittington and E. T. Beer
    1971   "Drug Use and Misuse Among the Elderly." *Journal of Drug Issues* 9:5–26.

Phillips, D. L., and B. E. Segal
    1969   "Sexual Status and Psychiatric Symptoms." *American Sociological Review* 34:58–72.

Pollin, W.
    1977   *Research on Smoking Behavior.* Washington: U.S. Government Printing Office.

Prehoda, R. W.
    1968   *Extended Youth: The Promise of Gerontology.* New York: Putnam's.

Roth, H. P., H. S. Caron, and B. P. Hsi
    1975   "Measuring Intake of a Prescribed Medication: A Bottle Count and Tracer Method Compared." *Clinical Pharmacological Therapy* 11:136–228.

Rothstein, M.
    1982   *Biochemical Approaches to Aging.* New York: Academic Press.

Royal College of Physicians of London
    1984   "Medication for the Elderly." *Journal of the Royal College of Physicians of London* 18(1):7–17.

Salzman, C. L.
    1982   "Basic Principles of Psychotropic Drug Prescriptions for the Elderly." *Hospital and Community Psychiatry* 33:133–36.

Schmeiser, D. A., H. W. B. Heumann, and J. R. Manning
    1974   *The Native Offender and the Law.* Ottawa: Law Reform Commission of Canada.

Schwartz, D., M. Wang, L. Zeitz, and E. W. Goss
    1962   "Medication Errors Made by the Elderly." *American Journal of Public Health* 52(12):2018–29.

Segerberg, Jr., O.
    1974   *The Immortality Factor.* New York: E. P. Dutton & Co.

Seidl, L. G., G. F. Thornton, J. W. Smith, and L. E. Cuff
    1966   "Studies on the Epidemiology of Adverse Drug Reactions." *Bulletin of Johns Hopkins Hospital* 119:229–315.

Shephard, R. J.
    1978   *Physical Activity and Aging.* London: Croom-Helm.

Shurtleff, D.
    1970   "Some Characteristics Related to the Incidence of Cardiovascular Disease and Death: Framingham Study, a 16 Year Follow-up." In W. B. Kannel and T. Gordon (eds.). *The Framingham Study,* Section 26. Washington, D.C.: U.S. Government Printing Office.

Simonson, W., and C. K. Sturgeon
  1979 "An Efficient Manual System to Increase Pharmacists' Ability to Detect and Prevent Medication Interactions." *Contemporary Pharmaceutical Practice* 2:175–80.
Skelton, D.
  1985 "Drug Utilization in a Relatively Fit Elderly Population." Paper Presented at the Canadian Association for Gerontology, Hamilton, Ontario.
Smith, E. L., and C. Gilligan
  1983 "Physical Activity Prescription for the Older Adult." *The Physician and Sports Medicine* 11:91–101.
Smith, M
  1976 "Portrayal of the Elderly in Prescription Drug Advertising." *The Gerontologist* 16:329–34.
Smith, P., and J. Andrews
  1983 "Drug Compliance not so Bad, Knowledge not so Good: The Elderly after Hospital Discharge." *Age and Aging* 12:336–42.
Spirduso, W. W.
  1980 "Physical Fitness, Aging and Psychomotor Speed: A Review." *Journal of Gerontology*, 36(6):850–65.
Stacey, C., A. Kozma, and M. J. Stones
  1985 "Simple Cognitive and Behavioral Changes Resulting from Improved Physical Fitness in Persons over 50 Years of Age." *Canadian Journal of Aging* 4(2):67–74.
Statistics Canada
  1983 *Apparent per Capita Food Consumption in Canada: Part I and Part II.* Ottawa: Statistics Canada.
  1984 *Canadian Women: Profile of Their Health.* (Catalogue No. 82-542E). Ottawa: Ministry of Supply and Services Canada.
Stephens, R. C., C. A. Hanley, and S. Underwood
  1981 "Psychoactive Drug Use and Potential Misuse among Persons Aged 55 Years and Older." *Journal of Psychoactive Drugs* 13(2):185–93.
Stewart, R. B., and L. E. Cluff
  1972 "A Review of Medication Errors and Compliance in Ambulant Patients." *Clinical Pharmacology and Therapeutics* 13(4):463–68.
Stones, M. J., and A. Kozma
  1985 "Physical Performance." In N. Charness (ed.). *Aging and Human Performance.* New York: John Wiley and Sons, Ltd.
Stones, M. J., A. Kozma, and L. Stones
  1985 "Preliminary Findings on the Effects of Exercise Program Participation in Older Adults." *Canadian Journal of Public Health* 76:272–73.
Stuchlikova, E., M. Juricova-Horakova, and Z. Deyl
  1975 "New Aspects of the Dietary Effects of Life Prolongation in Rodents. What is the Role of Obesity in Aging?" *Experimental Gerontology* 10:141–44.
Tannenbaum, A.
  1947 "The Effects of Varying Caloric Intake Upon Tumor Incidents and Tumor Growth." *Annals of the New York Academy of Science* 49:5–18.

Thompson, T. and C. R. Schuster
  1968 *Behavioral Pharmacology.* Englewood Cliffs, New Jersy: Prentice-Hall, Inc.

Thompson, H. T. L., M. G. Moran, and A. S. Nies
  1983 "Psychotropic Drug Use in the Elderly, Part I." New England *Journal of Medicine* 308:134–38.
  1983 "Psychotropic Drug Use in the Elderly, Part II." New England *Journal of Medicine* 308:194–98.

Trimmer, J.
  1967 *Rejuvenation: The History of an Idea.* New York: A. S. Barnes and Company.

Van Fraechem, J., and R. Van Fraechem
  1977 "Studies of the Effects of a Short Training Period on Aged Subjects." *Journal of Sports Medicine and Physical Fitness* 17:373–80.

Van Lancker, J. L.
  1977 "Smoking and Disease." In M. E. Jarvik, J. W. Cullen, E. R. Gritz and T. M. Vogt. *Research on Smoking and Behavior.* Washington: U.S. Government Printing Office.

Vanzant, F. R., W. C. Alvarez, G. B. Eusterman, H. L. Dunn and J. Bertson
  1932 "The Normal Range of Gastric Acidity for Youth to Old Age: An Analysis of 3,746 Records." *Archives of Internal Medicine* 47:345.

Vestal, R. E., E. A. McGuire, and J. D. Tobin, *et al.*
  1977 "Aging and Ethanol Metabolism." *Clinical Pharmacology and Therapy* 21:343–54.

Vischer, A. L.
  1947 *Old Age: Its Compensations and Rewards.* (trans. Bernard Miall). New York: The Macmillan Company.

Waldron, I.
  1977 "Increased Prescribing of Valium, Librium and Other Drugs: An Example of the Influence of Economic and Social Factors on the Practice of Medicine." *International Journal of Health Services* 7:62–73.

Walford, L.
  1983 *Maximum Life Span.* New York: W. W. Norton & Co.

Wallace, S., B. Whiting, and J. Runcie
  1976 "Factors Affecting Drug Binding in Plasma of Elderly Patients." *British Journal of Clinical Pharmacology* 3:327–30.

Wandless, I. and J. W. Davie
  1977 "Can Drug Compliance in the Elderly be Improved?" *British Medical Journal* 1:359–61.

Wasson, R.
  1968 *Soma, Divine Mushroom of Immortality.* New York: Harcourt Brace Jovanovich, Inc.

Whiting, B., and A. Goldberg
  1977 "The Use of the Drug Disc (MEDISC): A Warning System for Drug Interactions." In D. G. Grahame-Smith (ed.). *Drug Interactions.* Baltimore: University Park Press, 21–29.

Whittington, F. J.
  1979 "Drugs, Aging and Social Policy." In D. M. Peterson, F. J. Whittington

and B. P. Payne (eds.). *Drugs and the Elderly, Social and Pharmacological Issues*. Springfield, Illinois: Charles C. Thomas.

Whittington, F. J., D. M. Peterson, B. Dale, and P. L. Dressel
  1981 "Sex Differences in Prescription Drug Use of Older Adults." *Journal of Psychoactive Drugs* (2):175–83.

Williams, R. J.
  1973 *Nutrition Against Disease*. New York: Pitman.

Williamson, H., and J. M. Chopin
  1980 "Adverse Drug Reactions to Prescribed Drugs in the Elderly: A Multicentre Investigation." *Age and Aging* 9(2):73–80.

Winick, C.
  1962 "Maturing Out of Narcotic Addiction." *Bulletin on Narcotics* 14:1–7.

Wood, W. G.
  1985 "Mechanisms Underlying Age-related Differences in Response to Ethanol." In E. Gottheil, K. A. Druley, T. E. Skoloda and H. M. Waxman (eds.). *The Combined Problems of Alcoholism, Drug Addiction and Aging*. Springfield, Illinois: Charles C. Thomas.

Yano, K., G. G. Rhoads, and A. Kagan
  1977 "Coffee, Alcohol and Risk of Coronary Disease among Japanese Men Living in Hawaii." *New England Journal of Medicine* 297:405–409.

Zawadski, R. T., G. B. Glazer, and E. Laurie
  1978 "Psychotropic Drug Use Among Institutionalized and Noninstitutionalized Medicade Aged in California." *Journal of Gerontology* 33:825–34.

Zolier, M. L.
  1985 "Free Radicals: The Real Culprits in Aging?" *Geriatrics* 40(3):126–32.

Zwerling, I., R. Plutchik, M. Holtz, R. King, J. Crossman, and B. B. Siegel
  1975 "Effects of Procaine Preparations (Gerovital H3) in Hospital Geriatric Patients: A Double-bind study." *Journal of the American Geriatrics Society* 23:355–59.

INDEX